# STRAMONIUM

## With an Introduction to Analysis using Cycles and Segments

**Also by Paul Herscu, N.D.**

*The Homeopathic Treatment of Children:
Pediatric Constitutional Types*

# STRAMONIUM
## With an Introduction to Analysis using Cycles and Segments

### Paul Herscu, N.D.

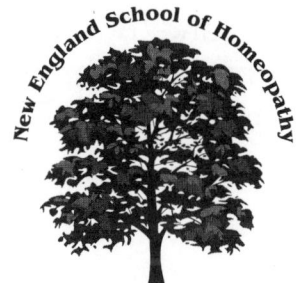

New England School of Homeopathy Press
Amherst, Massachusetts

# *Stramonium:*
## With an Introduction to Analysis using Cycles and Segments

Copyright © 1996 by Paul Herscu, N.D.
ISBN 0-9654004-0-9
All rights reserved

Published by
The New England School of Homeopathy Press
356 Middle Street, Amherst, Massachusetts 01002

Cover photograph by Steven Sloman
Steven Sloman Fine Arts, New York, New York
Index by S. Rosko Rossoff and Sequoia Cantin
Designed and Typeset by David Caputo

Printed in the United States of America

Copyright © 1996 by Paul Herscu, N.D. All rights reserved. No part of this book may be reproduced or transmitted in any form or by any means, electronic or mechanical, including photocopying, recording, or by any information storage and retrieval system, or otherwise without permission in writing from the publisher

This book is written as an educational resource for homeopathic physicians. It is not intended to replace appropriate diagnosis and/or treatment by a qualified physician. For information on the New England School of Homeopathy turn to page 187.

Published by
The New England School
of Homeopathy Press
356 Middle Street
Amherst, Massachusetts 01002
(413) 253-5949 • Fax: (413) 256-6223
www.nesh.com • nesh@nesh.com

Library of Congress Catalog Card Number: 96-70061
ISBN 0-9654004-0-9

*This book is dedicated to all children who suffer on deep levels
and the patient, loving people who take care of them.*

*It is also dedicated to all who practice homeopathy.
May we all be blessed with the good fortune of
seeing the right patient at the right time,
with clarity of vision, and occasionally
with divine inspiration.*

# Acknowledgments

A new book hits the market. The author's name there on the cover says, "I wrote this." But in truth, so many people go into the creation of a book. Below are the names of many people without whom *Stramonium* would not have been possible. I would like to express my appreciation and gratitude to them for their contributions. I know that for them, as for myself, the greatest reward will be whatever healing this book can bring to those who are suffering.

Special thanks to Amy Rothenberg, ND, my wife and partner with whom I practice, who contributed thirty cases of *Stramonium* to help confirm my own data and observations. Beside the contribution of the cases, Amy greatly helped in the refinement of concepts presented in this book. But more importantly, she gave unending love to me and our children, which ultimately allowed for this work to be born.

Peggy Chipkin, RN, FNP, Durr Elmore, DC, ND, Vassilis Ghegas, MD, Alan Greenberg, DC, George Guess, MD, Nancy Herrick, PA, Robert Israel, MD, Paul Mittman, ND, Randall Neustaedter, OMD, Nicholas Nossaman, MD, Jeremy Sherr, FSHom, Jonathan Shore, MD, Ilene Spector, DO, and Michael Thompson, FSHom, who generously sent forty-eight of the cases included in this volume.

Micki Elia, for typing the original manuscript.

Elizabeth Powers, Iain Marrs, and Lauri Grossman, DC, who initially edited portions of the book.

Jeenet Lawton, who as chief editor, was a pleasure to work with, and shared invaluable insight into the art of writing. As a homeopath, she also provided constant feedback as to how a student of homeopathy would perceive the text, and pushed me to further clarify my ideas.

Steven Sloman, whose homeopathic understanding of the remedy led to his artistic interpretation, which graces the cover of this book.

S. Rosco Rossoff, for his comprehensive index.

David Caputo, for a beautiful layout design, concept, and execution.

Alice Duncan, DC, for proofreading the final text.

Durr Elmore DC, ND, and Frank Gruber, MD, who provided an immense amount of moral support for my work, as well as proofreading the final text.

Mary Ann Dietschler, who has greatly supported my efforts, and the growth of the New England School of Homeopathy, for the past four years.

Abraham and Clara Herscu, my parents who have always supported me in love and spirit.

# Table of Contents

Acknowledgements . . . . . . . . . . . . . . . . . . . . . . . . . . . . . . . . . . . . . viii
Foreword. . . . . . . . . . . . . . . . . . . . . . . . . . . . . . . . . . . . . . . . . . . . . . . xi
Author's Comments . . . . . . . . . . . . . . . . . . . . . . . . . . . . . . . . . . . . xiii

## Part One: New Ideas Need a New Language

Cycles . . . . . . . . . . . . . . . . . . . . . . . . . . . . . . . . . . . . . . . . . . . . . . . . 3
*A new model of understanding the materia medica*

The Map of Hierarchy . . . . . . . . . . . . . . . . . . . . . . . . . . . . . . . . . . 15
*A description of a predictable order of remedies a patient may need over time*

The *Stramonium* Cycle . . . . . . . . . . . . . . . . . . . . . . . . . . . . . . . . . 27

A Whole Book on *Stramonium*? . . . . . . . . . . . . . . . . . . . . . . . . . 37

## Part Two: The Materia Medica of *Stramonium*

### Mind
Fear . . . . . . . . . . . . . . . . . . . . . . . . . . . . . . . . . . . . . . . . . . . . . 43
Violence . . . . . . . . . . . . . . . . . . . . . . . . . . . . . . . . . . . . . . . . 69
Attention Difficulties . . . . . . . . . . . . . . . . . . . . . . . . . . . . . 89
Introversion . . . . . . . . . . . . . . . . . . . . . . . . . . . . . . . . . . . . . 99
Autism . . . . . . . . . . . . . . . . . . . . . . . . . . . . . . . . . . . . . . . . 105

Sleep . . . . . . . . . . . . . . . . . . . . . . . . . . . . . . . . . . . . . . . . . . . . 115

Body . . . . . . . . . . . . . . . . . . . . . . . . . . . . . . . . . . . . . . . . . . . . 135

## Appendix
Aphorisms . . . . . . . . . . . . . . . . . . . . . . . . . . . . . . . . . . . . . . 181
New England School of Homeopathy . . . . . . . . . . . . . . . . 187

Index . . . . . . . . . . . . . . . . . . . . . . . . . . . . . . . . . . . . . . . . . . . . . . 189

# *Foreword*

I am very happy that Paul Herscu has dedicated a book to *Stramonium*, which will increase the awareness for this remedy. The more one studies homeopathy, the more one realizes that there are many facets to each remedy. The material written in the old books, while very good, only represents one view of a remedy and usually emphasizes the extreme pathologic picture. In the old *Stramonium* material we read about wildness, violence, and delusions. If that were all that we prescribed upon, we would have to wait until the *Stramonium* patients were very ill before we could find help for them.

Unfortunately, the material to replace these older books is only now being published, including my *Materia Medica Viva*. Because of this lack of information, since many people learn only the extreme form of individual remedies, they are not able to recognize the seemingly healthy and less severely compromised states. For instance, the materia medica lists *Stramonium* as very reactive, very violent, and with strong neurologic symptoms, yet many patients do not fit these extreme descriptions. Dr. Herscu's book should go a long way toward fine tuning the symptoms that relate to the entire range of *Stramonium*.

One of the best personal experiences I encountered to demonstrate this point was the case of a woman in England suffering with lymphoma. Some of her symptoms were abdominal pain, with mucousy stools that alternated between constipation and diarrhea. She liked sweets and vegetables and disliked meat. She was timid, shy, sensitive, mild, sentimental, lacked confidence and was very neat. She had fears of pins and of being alone and had had a terrible disappointment in her love life. She had vertigo from high places.

Many of the conference participants saw *Pulsatilla* quite strongly and wanted to prescribe it, as it was the obvious choice. Yet the Vithoulkas Expert System kept on coming up with *Stramonium*. I gave *Stramonium* and it acted beautifully; the patient was cured, went on to have a wonderful pregnancy and baby. The point here is that the participants could not see *Stramonium* because they did not see in front of them the extreme form of the remedy. This book should make it easier to find *Stramonium* when the patient is not in that extreme form.

This above mentioned case also illustrates one of the main points of this book. Understanding *Stramonium* in its relationship to other remedies can help us in our practice to give the needed remedy at the right time.

George Vithoulkas

# Author's Comments

The introduction is often thought of as the part of the book to skip over, a tedious trek through the author's brain, telling you all the things he thinks may not be clear in the book.

So right now I am inviting you to skip PART ONE if you are eager to get to the materia medica of *Stramonium*. *But please come back later*. You are going to see *Stramonium* as you've not seen it before, and this section tells you why. Not only is it *Stramonium* that is put under the microscope, but also the very way we look at remedies.

Two different groups of people have shaped my approach to treating patients, studying remedies and making prescriptions:

First, the thousands of children I have personally seen in my practice, as well as those I have heard about from colleagues who have helped shape what was missing from the materia medica for this type of child. There are a lot of children out there nowadays who just do not fit the good old polychrests. But our information in the old materia medicas about the more emotionally or mentally challenged remedies is often misleading or incomplete, especially regarding children. So it is these children themselves who showed me what was missing from the materia medicas.

Second, the fifteen hundred or so homeopaths I have listened to and taught throughout the United States and Europe, who have showed me what was missing in the teaching and helped me to hone the information into an accessible and understandable form.

And so it all just sort of happened. This book is the second of several that has grown out of my personal experience as a student, physician and teacher.

I'm excited! I'm thinking about the way things were and how they've changed and what we have to do next. I'm thinking about *how remedies work*, not just about keynotes or mental symptoms. And I'm thinking that there's got to be an easier, faster, more effective way of eliciting the case history as well as studying and understanding remedies.

# STRAMONIUM

Above all, this book is a shot into the future. The ideas represented in PART ONE are not meant to be complete, but rather to open avenues of dialogue and exploration, as well as to place into context the materia medica of *Stramonium*. PART TWO contains the materia medica of *Stramonium*. Unlike other materia medicas, this one attempts to keep tying the symptoms to the main ideas (segments of the cycle) they belong to.

From time to time I come across something in literature or poetry which elicits in me something of the feeling of a particular remedy. Scattered throughout these pages are a few selections which created in me a kinesthetic sense of *Stramonium*. My hope is that they will help to create in the reader a semblance of the mood one might feel while taking a *Stramonium* case.

One last point. To avoid the use of he/she language in the materia media, I decided to describe the remedy only in the masculine gender. Another reason I did this is that most of children that are described in this book happen to be boys. When a particular point relates more to girls, it is designated as such.

***

Homeopathy is growing so fast that we have to catch up with it. I'm inviting you to come along with me on a journey that started over two hundred years ago, and is now as exciting and innovative as it was then.

# Part One
## New Ideas Need a New Language

# *Cycles*

Some two hundred years ago a great adventure began. A brilliant and creative physician whose motto was *Be bold and be sensible* dared to question the medical establishment. Faced with certain practices in medicine that did not make sense to him, Samuel Hahnemann started out to find the *why* behind the healing action of a single drug, and ended up taking a giant leap in uncovering the link between drugs and diseases.

In my mind Samuel Hahnemann was to medicine what Sir Isaac Newton was to physics. Both offered us a new way of thinking and new laws to match it. Both developed their views by incorporating old theories, observations, and experiential data, and both came up with universal concepts that explained aspects of nature. Newton's models and rules enhanced our understanding of how things work—things that we observe every day, such as gravity and the movement of the planets. Similarly, Hahnemann's ideas explained the why of ordinary things—why people become sick and why certain symptoms manifest.

Using Newton's theories, it was possible to accurately predict phenomena that would not be discovered or understood for two hundred years. Similarly, Hahnemann's theory of miasms and disease foreshadowed the discovery of germs, bacteria, and viruses.

Both men's theories contain certain assumptions, assumptions that hold those theories together and allow for them to exist in the first place. Newton proposed that space and time were continuous and constant and that we move through a thing called *aether*. Hahnemann proposed that the 'symptom' was, is, always will be, and in fact, *must be* the tool to match the patient to the remedy.

These great men's universal concepts helped us to better understand things we observe in our daily life. However, both theories failed to answer certain nagging questions. Newton's theory regarding constants was challenged by the electromagnetic experiments of the late nineteenth century and the observations regarding the speed of light. Hahnemann's theory of basing our prescription on the symptom has served us well, but it has also generated some problems and controversy. The problem that concerns me most is the somewhat haphazard manner of deciding which symptoms to base a prescription on and the confusion that this generates.

## A New Model

People use mental models to explain how things work. The model is not reality, it is simply one way of describing how we see reality, based upon the totality of our observations and experiences. As we add to our understanding, we often need to refine our models to reflect this new view of reality.

Today a new model is needed, a model that reflects the new insights in homeopathy, a model that can:

- explain all the old phenomena
- incorporate and explain all the new phenomena
- predict with accuracy future phenomena

This model must help us to understand both the totality of the patient and the totality of the remedy, as well as help us decide how to approach the analysis of the patient.

When we first begin studying homeopathy, we learn about matching the totality of the whole person with the totality of the remedy. This is the 'party line'. But in actual practice we begin to discover that this is not so easy. At first we try to use *all* of the symptoms, but then we end up with a mass of confusion and errors. Puzzled, we scratch our heads and tentatively shift into using only a part of the total case. That forces us to choose *which* part. Which symptoms will lead to success? Which to failure? And how do we go about choosing? At this point, many of us fall back on aphorism #153 of the *Organon*, "…the most striking, strange, unusual, peculiar signs and symptoms in the case are especially, almost exclusively, the ones to which close attention should be given…" And by making this choice, we settle for a middle ground. We are no longer paying attention to the whole patient, but rather to a part (what Stuart Close called the 'logical' totality).

# CYCLES

By shifting into analyzing only a part of the total case, we inadvertently shift into a gray zone. But, as in all gray zones, there are difficulties to contend with. When things are not black and white, when there is room for interpretations and options, then there is also an opening for miscalculations. One homeopath will choose one set of symptoms, another will choose a different set. Then to support our choice, we try to make an argument for this mental symptom or that keynote or this physical general. But we are not completely convinced. We fumble and stumble and wonder if we will ever get the hang of it.

Then someone pats us on the back and says, "As you gain more experience, it will be easier for you to choose the correct set of symptoms." And even though there may be some truth in that, it is a kind of reverse logic. After all, how helpful is it to tell someone that the more homeopathy you know and the more experience you have, the easier it will be to maneuver in the gray zones and the more likely your choice of symptoms will be correct? This is what beginning homeopaths have been told all too often.

But wait a minute. How about the patients who are not getting well in the meantime? Not only do they lose out, but the beginning homeopath has lost some of his zest and is experiencing anxiety, frustration, and insecurity instead of the excitement and joy that should be his.

Does this mean that the art of homeopathy can only be mastered by a few? Not at all. It simply means that we have to reexamine the thinking behind the teaching models we have been using and find new models, new methods that will make the homeopath's first steps smaller, less harsh, and more rewarding. Granted that this book presents my way, and I think it is a sound way, but it is not the only way. I believe there are numerous answers to these problems, and all of us need to be searching for them. We each see the world differently, and by making the best of those differences, we could all come up with many new ways to look at problems and create solutions. As they say, it wouldn't have been the Swing Era if only Benny Goodman played. To create a movement, a science, we must all participate.

It does not matter which solutions you personally choose to follow and to create. What does matter is that we continue to search for and find something less limiting than what exists at the present time, something that will enhance our ability to prescribe more successfully and to end more suffering.

# STRAMONIUM

Maybe this is a good time to share with you the ideas that helped me tackle this problem and resolve it for myself.

## Watching the drama of the Vital Force

I thought about how we come into the world with a body and spirit and our vital force. It animates us and, in a sense, *is* us. But the health of that vital force will vary from one person to the next. From the moment of our conception, it is affected by various genetic as well as environmental factors. Then along comes a stress that the person is susceptible to, and the vital force is overwhelmed and knocked out of balance. And that's how disease begins.

Disease is a unit. It is one disease for one person at one time. It begins in a single place (usually the individual's weakest spot) but it also shows itself throughout the whole being in many ways, manifesting through many signposts which we call signs and symptoms. Our job is to ferret out that *one* disease for that one person. The vital force's job is to help us find it, by producing signs, or symptoms, that show us the pattern of the disease.

How does the vital force do this? When it first gets 'untuned', it *strains* to adjust to the stress, in order to reestablish its balance. This straining is what produces the symptoms that point out the disorder and signal what is wrong. Another way of putting it is that the vital force, thrown off balance by the stress, no longer has the ability to cure. It is flawed. Its efforts fail. This failed attempt is itself the chronic disease illustrated in full color. Thus, the symptoms are not the disorder itself but in some way show the disorder, by mirroring it or embodying it.

How can we best see the message that the vital force is struggling so hard to show us? It is flashing the pathology of the whole patient at us, if only we could see it. Its message can be detected in every symptom of the patient. That is the genius of the vital force. It is doing a great job. If, by giving us dozens or maybe hundreds of examples, the vital force can say in a nutshell, "This is it. This is the disease," why can't we? What a help it would be if we could describe with a single statement every symptom that a remedy can produce or cure.

But there is a nagging question getting in the way. *If there is only one disease, how do **all** the symptoms fit together?* Not just *most* of the symptoms, not just the ones we selected, but *all* of the symptoms, the mental state, the sleep position, the food cravings and aversions, the common as well as the characteristic symptoms.

Until now, we have been forced to settle for the bulk of the symptoms and let go of the rest. We have learned several mechanistic models of understanding, and by trial and error eventually found success more and more. But here comes that nagging again: Why not *every* symptom? If the disease is throughout the being, then every single symptom, from unimportant ones to important ones, should in some way *mirror that disease*. So what can we do? We need to understand and match not just the symptoms of the illness, but—more importantly—the *way* of being sick. How can we go about doing that?

## Another Voice

As T.S. Eliot said in his *Four Quartets*, "...next year's words await another voice." I am struck by the fact that, although our profession has a strong vitalistic philosophy, the practical application has often been mechanical at best. So, if we hope to create a more practical, effective, streamlined way of case taking and repertorization, we need to find new words for saying what we have to say and new ways of saying it.

A number of homeopaths, including myself, have been working on developing a universal method of studying and practicing homeopathy. Using a common language, this method could act as a matrix within which classical homeopaths can express their different ways of teaching, prescribing, and writing. By so doing, they can add to each other's findings, thereby refining homeopathy and propelling it forward. What follows is my initial contribution to this pool of knowledge.

I have been working on a way that I think will allow us to easily and succinctly describe a remedy. It involves formulating a phrase or sentence for each remedy that will fit *every symptom* of that remedy, *every patient* we have ever seen who needed that remedy, fit *every materia medica* we have read, *every lecture* we have heard, and *every live case* as well as *paper cases* we have studied of that remedy. It must be a precise statement that sums up not only all that this remedy encapsulates, but *also the dynamic aspect* of it, how it moves from one stage of the illness to the next. For *Stramonium* such a sentence might be: **Driven by confusion, fears, and vulnerability, *Stramonium* is engaged in an ongoing and violent battle between the unconscious and the conscious, between darkness and light, between succumbing to the death realm and yearning to exist in the life realm.** Examined carefully, everything about *Stramonium* should fit this picture. But more of that in the *Stramonium Cycle* section.

If we can begin to understand each remedy in the materia medica in this way, there will be much less need to memorize facts and facts and facts. Why? Because this kind of learning leads to understanding. Why should we settle for memorizing when we can understand?

Would this enhanced way of looking at remedies and patients contradict what Hahnemann taught us? Not in the least. It is quite in line with the picture Hahnemann painted—a picture of the vital force putting on a show (for the purpose of preserving the patient). The vital force *strains* to shout out the plot. The symptoms are the main characters, not just bit players entering and exiting in some haphazard fashion. They move within a script in a logical pattern. It is this logical pattern that homeopaths have been trying to perceive all along.

I believe this pattern is what Hahnemann meant when he spoke about a *totality of symptoms*. By totality he did not simply mean the total number of symptoms, but rather the *total pattern* of the disease. That is the real totality. I do not see the pattern as being just mental or emotional or physical. It is a pattern of unfolding. It does not begin or end at any one point.

What is that unfolding, or movement?

- The vital force gets knocked off center by some stress.
- To correct that and reestablish a balance, it *strains*.
- The strain shows itself in signs and symptoms.
- These symptoms grow stronger as the vital force compensates too much, until they finally overshoot the mark.
- The overshoot must be corrected to maintain some semblance of balance.
- That, in time, brings the patient full cycle back to (or at least near to) where he started.

# CYCLES

In this way the cycle is reinforced, over and over again. It is as if you are getting on a train, trying to go directly to a certain destination. But the train instead makes a loop, stopping at various places along that loop and finally coming back to where you first began. This loop or cycle is the disease, and it keeps repeating itself over and over again. We will see this later in the Cycle of *Stramonium*.

How can the cycle ever be broken? A shift is needed in the underlying balance so that the patient can return to health. But change is hard to come by; it is easier to go on and on in the rut of the cycle. If you reflect upon your own life, you may recall times when you found yourself in somewhat of a 'stuck' mode, and you struggled to get free of it, but the more you tried to break the pattern or habit, the deeper you went into the rut.

The fluid action of chronic disease is like that. It first establishes a certain pattern and then renews itself by falling into the same groove over and over again, each time sinking deeper, spiraling downward. The deterioration shows up in the mental and emotional and physical spheres in different ways. This pattern, this cycle of events, will (in some way) be recognizable everywhere—in all the symptoms of the patient, in all the symptoms listed in the materia medica for that remedy, and in all the symptoms brought out in the provings.

If we can look at disease in this way, we will be better able to identify and isolate the main elements or ideas, which I call **fundamental segments,** within each of the remedies. That will allow us to recreate the chain of events showing the pattern that fits not only everything known about that remedy, but everything known about every patient who has ever needed it. It will even give us the freedom to predict the direction the disease will take.

## The Fundamental Segments within the Cycle

*Everything* you are looking at in your patient is showing the same balancing act of the vital force. Believe it. Look for it.

**I sincerely believe that every single symptom a person expresses is an example of one of the fundamental segments operating in that person's cycle of disease.** This includes even our strong symptoms, our mental symptoms, our sleep symptoms, everything. Each one is an *example*. This

## STRAMONIUM

explains why we get in trouble when we take the keynotes literally. That is, we think the person *must* desire sweets in order to fit *Stramonium*. But sweets is only an example of the yearning for comfort in this isolated and lonely person. In other words, a symptom does not stand alone. It has a relationship of some kind to other symptoms. And so, that desire for comfort or consolation, which is one of the fundamental segments of the remedy, will show up over and over again in many places and many ways through various symptoms. Some of these symptoms will be found in rubrics; some will not. That doesn't matter. It is the segment, the idea, that matters. That segment is something which absolutely belongs to that remedy.

**The cycle itself is a flow of events that is composed of a number of fundamental segments.** Each one of these segments could be described by a word or phrase, such as *yearning for comfort* or *violent overreactions*. In the model showing the cycle, you will see that each segment is linked by an arrow to the next segment, representing its direct effect leading to the one that follows. It in some way pushes the person to the next segment. Each segment flows into the next until you come full cycle again. *The cycle is the disease.* You can jump in at any point, start with any segment. The pattern is a continuous flow.

Another way of looking at it: Picture for a moment a circle of stepping stones surrounding a flower bed. A different cluster of flowers is planted next to each stone. As you move from one stone to the next, you see a whole new cluster. Each is part of the total design. At some point you return to the original cluster. In the cycle of a remedy, these clusters are the fundamental segments of the cycle.

To stretch the metaphor a bit further, different flowers are planted and bloom and die at different times, and there may be others to come up in their place. Similarly, the disease is not stationary but continuously flowing, moving, and changing—but only within certain parameters. One thing is sure—every item that appears in a materia medica must in some way fit into one of those idea clusters, or segments, that make up the total pattern of the remedy. This is why I call it a **fundamental segment**—*fundamental* because it is intrinsic and essential; *segment* because it is a part of the whole cycle.

Another point. Within every remedy you will see certain segments that seem universal, such as weakness. At first this may seem confusing. How can you differentiate between dozens of remedies if they all have segments in common? Easily. *The uniqueness of that remedy will be apparent in specifically **how** that element or segment (weakness) is expressed.* Also every remedy will have at least one segment that is unique unto itself.

However, every symptom of the remedy is not unique and we cannot treat it as such, for the vital force is not split in pieces. It strains as one, it reacts as one, and it must be seen as one. This point was made clear to me eight years ago when a pregnant woman called saying that as soon as she washed her face she began to bleed from the vagina. Now there is no rubric like 'threatened miscarriage from washing the face'. But there is one saying that washing the face causes a nosebleed. So I thought, "Well, if bathing can cause bleeding in one place, why can't it cause it anywhere? The location is secondary to the bleeding and to the modality. The remedy chosen, *Arnica montana*, stopped the miscarriage and the child was born healthy. This same principle has been applied to babies who after birth have an epileptic fit when bathed and later are shown to have had a bleed within the brain.

**So, at times it is possible, even useful, to generalize a symptom.** Boenninghausen was the first to state this point clearly. It is the job of the homeopath to do this kind of generalizing, grouping all symptoms into segments or units that make sense. In most remedies there will be found four to six fundamental segments. Each of these can be broken down into smaller segments, giving even more flavor to the remedy. For example, in the *Stramonium* cycle presented here, I chose to make hyperactivity into a subsection of the violent overreaction segment.

*Once you understand these clusters of ideas that belong to a remedy, you will easily be able to predict other symptoms that might fit under one segment or another. And you will also be able to predict with some accuracy the rubrics that the remedy should be found in.* You can see how such an innovative tool would be invaluable in checking your findings as you never could before.

## Which Symptoms Go Under Which Segment?

The tough part at first is learning how to figure out which rubrics to group together to form each segment in the cycle. Some of the segments will be easier than others to work with. For example, take three different symptoms: a *cramp in the abdomen, a cramp in the calf, a twitch in the toe*. Although they are in different locations, they are similar in the *idea of cramping*. So it is easy to see that cramping will be one of the fundamental segments for this patient.

Of course, different homeopaths perceive things differently. Some look for similarities, some look for differences. Some will see *cramping* and *twitching* as similar. Some will see them as different. Some will see *cramping* and *obstinacy* as similar. That is less obvious. What if you have *cramping* and *twitching* and *constipation*? What do they have in common? *Contraction*. What about *constipation, cramping* and *obstinacy*? This shows that they all are *holding on to things*. Even though all these symptoms represent the same idea, some will see that and others may not.

Sooner or later you will have a patient who is *sensitive to light, touch* and *noise*, and you will see that what these symptoms have in common is *sensitivity*. Less obvious but also similar would be *sensitivity to noise, aversion to touch*, and *fear of robbers*. Are these similar? Yes, they all represent *fear of invasion*. It is almost uncanny how much you can predict with this form of assessing. *Not only can you predict symptoms you will find in the patient, but even symptoms you will find in the materia medica.*

Some of the fundamental segments or groupings will be more abstract than others. Those will be harder to perceive at first. For instance, what do the following have in common: *desire to be rubbed, desires consolation, desire to be carried*? *Comfort*. That one was easy. But what about *desire for milk, sweets, pies, ice cream, and fruit*? Actually all of them are *comfort foods*, the kind of foods we seek when we want comforting or when there's an issue of being forsaken. So you have a patient who is ameliorated by consolation, but when you look up that rubric the remedy you feel is correct is not there. Every homeopath eventually faces this—finding good rubrics that do not contain the correct remedy. What then? What can you do? Look at the patient's food cravings—one happens to be sweets, a comfort signal. You choose that, simply because you can see in it the same segment you find running throughout, that same emotion of yearning for comfort. And here's where predicting comes in. I guarantee that you will find many other symptoms in that patient which represent the same idea. That same idea must be there, everywhere, because it is a fundamental segment.

# CYCLES

Another thing that can be frustrating is getting a great symptom that is rare and peculiar, but there's no rubric for it. How often has that happened to you? Or you find the rubric for that peculiar symptom but, lo and behold, the remedy you expect to be there is not (as in the comfort example above). Then what can you do? The cycle of the segments is a way of solving some of these common problems.

## The Flow of the Cycle

Once we see the relationship of a number of symptoms such as *desires consolation, craves sweets, pain better from touch, and ear pain better from being carried,* then we have understood one of the fundamental segments in the patient's cycle. Next we have to find out what events caused this to arise in the first place. How did this *need for comforting* come into being? And what keeps it functioning? And after we have understood where it came from, the next question is where does it lead the patient? What does it make him do next? The answer to these questions will lead you right into the next segment. Perhaps his need for comfort and consolation makes him overshoot and go into excessive behaviors, outbursts, or some other form of overreaction. If so, you will find similar ideas in the body symptoms that will belong to this group. If the excesses (in this patient) then lead to *exhaustion*, you have now moved into another segment. And so it goes from one idea to the next to the next, until you come full cycle. At this point the whole cycle will be clear to you.

Your job, as a homeopath, is to keep figuring out how and why each segment leads to something else, or even moves on to a different pathology, but one that shows the same issues, the same elements. You can find a more complete example in *The Stramonium Cycle*.

These patterns are patterns of the whole person, not just of the mind or the emotions or the body. Some of your patients will show you the pattern and even tell it in the sequence that matters to them. Other cases will not be so easy because the symptoms may seem so far apart, making it harder to see what they have in common.

For example, I once treated a woman who said, *"I have thoracic pain that feels like someone is poking at my back...I am afraid of crowds...I like to sit on the aisle...I lock the doors at night."* All of these symptoms contain an element of suspiciousness, a feeling of mistrust or doubt, an idea that something is wrong. Even the back pain fits that idea. So it was no surprise to me when I was about to give her a remedy that it was necessary to spend another fifteen minutes talking about the remedy and about homeopathy, because of her suspicious nature. You see how predictable it was?

These main ideas that cycle around are the most important thing to look for in the patient. They cycle around, one after another popping up to show you the pathology. They *are* the pathology. Once you have seen these main ideas or fundamental segments, your next job is to arrange the bulk of the symptoms under each segment. The history and analysis are over and it is time to repertorize.

**Looking Toward the Future**

This is the job of the materia medicas of the future. We need this type of materia medica that can explain the whole picture of the pathology. Even though I have published several articles showing the cycles of certain remedies, this book is my first complete description of the totality of a remedy. Among these pages you hopefully will find answers to *why* the *Stramonium* child becomes fearful or develops violence, and *what it leads him to next*.

We are at a turning point in homeopathy, moving from the materia medicas of the past to those of the future. In the past it was the symptom that was emphasized. In the future we will be looking with more interest at the ideas behind the symptoms. Why do these particular symptoms exist in the first place? Where do they come from? What do they lead to?

In a time of transition, *Stramonium* is a transition book. What better remedy to make a bow as a transition book than one which bridges the gap between the polychrests and miasms and the phase four remedies, one which is in itself a transitional remedy in the **Map of Hierarchy.**

# The Map of Hierarchy

The cycle helps us to see the intrinsic qualities and the dynamic flow of the patient's illness. But there is still another issue facing us. Many of these children who are violent, impulsive, or have attention difficulties tend to exhibit symptoms and states that are so similar that selecting a remedy is often difficult. The confusion does not stop there. These children tend to exhibit symptoms of several remedies at the same time, and this forces us to meander through a maze, trying to figure out which one of the remedies is the correct choice. We need a map to guide us through this maze, a map that will help us to select the right symptoms to prescribe upon. Why is this issue so important? Because these children tend to have symptoms that are so similar, it has led us to mistakenly assume that all of those children need the same remedy. For instance, we may think that all violent kids need *Stramonium* or all hyperactive kids need *Veratrum album*, and so forth. To complicate the situation further, the different remedies that address these disorders also have many similar symptoms. No wonder the diligent homeopath has such a hard time determining the right remedy for such children. The remedies look so alike, one thinks that any of them could be used for these problems.

To add to the confusion, in the existing materia medicas there is only a sketchy description of the remedies most often used for the disorders we see today. What we read mostly refers to either acute pathologic states such as infection or to severe neurologic disorders or insanity. That was the information which applied to the patients of the era when these books were written.

So, the homeopath of today, in possession of confusing, inaccurate, and incomplete information, faces quite a challenge in finding the exact remedy for children with attention or impulse disorders. It is all too often beyond the scope of what is known and written. Thus it becomes a chore to decipher the old books so that we can find something applicable in today's world.

While homeopathy has helped us to achieve many brilliant successes with a number of these children, the aforementioned difficulties have led us to fail with many others who could have been cured had we taken a different approach. Faced with such difficult choices myself, I began sorting through numerous cases and observations. These led me to create what I call the **Map of Hierarchy.** This map enables us to understand why remedy states occur in the order they do for any individual child over time. It lays out remedies commonly used for these children, and the relationship between the remedies. At the same time that I realized how much need there was for updated materia medica information, I could see that it was equally important to develop a new approach to that information, a new way to differentiate these remedies, a way that would cut through the confusion of layers and symptoms and help to guide the practitioner toward the remedy needed at any given time.

The following model, the Map of Hierarchy, is what I came up with. I have been teaching it for the past six years, as a way of differentiating between the groups of remedies that seem to work well for children with behavior, learning and attention difficulties.

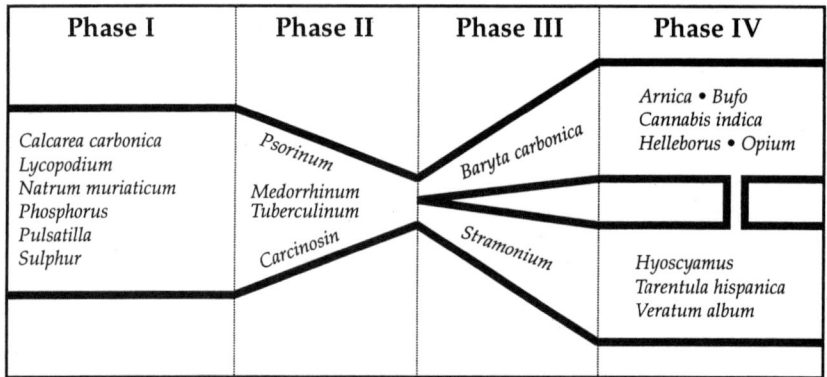

## The Map of Hierarchy

Basically, I believe that all remedies on this grid are not equal in the following respect: each phase represents a deeper state of pathology, progressing from left to right. Phase two is worse than phase one, phase three is worse than phase two, and phase four is worse than phase three. Thus the four phases are not equal in intensity.

It is not surprising then that the remedies in each phase follow the same rule. They also are not equal. *Medorrhinum's* state is worse than

## THE MAP OF HIERARCHY

*Calcarea carbonica's*, *Stramonium's* state is worse than *Medorrhinum's*, and *Hyoscyamus* is sicker than *Stramonium*. In saying this, I am **deliberately** placing a value judgment on the remedy itself and even on the state of the remedy. I do this as an innovation, and at first it may seem an unlikely thing to do. But it is not new in the sense of departing from the old. In a way, it is not really new to homeopathy. The same idea is inherent in Hering's Law—that there is a direction of cure, a *direction* in which the patient should travel as he becomes healthy. The main difference here is that we are looking at whole remedies in relation to each other instead of only symptoms in relation to each other.

Over the years, many homeopaths observed that as patients became healthier they tended to travel from one remedy state to another, but the process always seemed haphazard and confusing. Why the need for a change in remedies? Had they made a mistake? This shifting of remedies only caused more confusion and made the case go awry.

However, if we look at the whole patient population of children (as opposed to any individual child), we see that as they get healthier, they travel from deeper states to more superficial states, directly from phase four to phase one, or from phase three to phase one, or from the fourth phase to the third, then to the second, and finally to the first. One thing is consistent, they travel from the right part of the diagram toward the left. Of course, there are exceptions, such as a shock that sends someone speedily from the first phase back into the third. *We see in our practice, time and again, that the sicker these children become, the more they tend to need remedies in the fourth phase and that the healthier they become, the more they need remedies in the first phase. Further,* **given symptoms that are equal in duration and intensity,** *the symptoms that fit the third or fourth phase will be more pathologic than those in the first and second.* For example, even though both *Pulsatilla* and *Hyoscyamus* have the symptom of jealousy, *Hyoscyamus* is a more pathologic state because the symptom potential of *Hyoscyamus* is worse than the symptom potential of *Pulsatilla*. In other words, each remedy is not just a collection of symptoms, but a potential for future disease. It is this that gives us a hierarchy for the remedies.

So really it was by observing the process of healing that the Map of Hierarchy came to me, not from philosophical reflection or theorizing. In a way, it shows us Hering's Law operating on a larger scale, with whole remedies (instead of merely symptoms) moving in a direction either toward healing or toward deeper pathology.

If this is so, then this Map of Hierarchy provides us with a relatively easy way to match *the deepest pathology that exists at any one time*, thus applying Hahnemann's dictate to treat what has to be treated now, to match the deepest pathology first. Hopefully it will add a new depth to the way we select remedies.

To summarize the Map of Hierarchy: Given the choice between two remedies, if the two seem equal in intensity, it is best to treat with the remedy that fits the deeper phase. If you must choose between *Medorrhinum* and *Stramonium*, it is usually best to give *Stramonium*. And if you have an equal choice between *Stramonium* and *Hyoscyamus*, then give *Hyoscyamus*. What you are essentially doing is treating the deeper state first (as defined by the grid and the remedies found within the grid).

Let me add here that I want this map to be a help, not a hindrance. The remedies listed in each phase are only presented as examples, as possibilities, and should guide you rather than limit you. Please do not consider the list of remedies to be final. It is not complete and can never really be complete. You can add to these categories on the basis of your own experiences. The map is not the territory, it is a way of understanding the progress or decline of a patient's health.

Why do I place certain remedies in the different grid locations? Let us take a brief look at each phase and examine why the remedies are placed in their particular locations.

**Phase one fits the remedies that have to do with everyday constitutional needs of the patient.** The larger polychrests fit in here. For this group of remedies it almost does not matter which symptoms you choose. You could look only at food cravings, or only at the mental/emotional symptoms or only at the physical generals or only at the keynotes. No matter how you look at the case, most likely you will find the correct remedy. These are usually the cases we begin our practices with, and the great results we get lead us to think that homeopathy is a cinch.

**Phase two fits the nosodes.** These are special remedies in several ways. One way they may act is simply as a remedy layer, just as any other remedy

## THE MAP OF HIERARCHY

does. They clearly show themselves with all the symptoms, the mentals and emotionals, the keynotes, and the physical generals, just like any remedy in the first phase. *However, there is another possibility—that the nosode may not show itself as a unique remedy layer all at one time. Sometimes the nosodes will appear to be intertwined with some underlying remedy. In such a case you will see not just one remedy but hints of two.* You may see *Sulphur* intertwined with *Medorrhinum* or perhaps *Calcarea carbonica* mixed with *Tuberculinum*. There will be clear symptoms for both remedies at the same time, and that makes the choice even harder and the results less predictable. This is one of the unique aspects of the nosodes.

There is a second, more universal, point. As a child moves from the first phase to the second, he retains some or many of the symptoms belonging to the first phase. This means that any *Medorrhinum* or *Tuberculinum* child will also have symptoms of another remedy such as *Lycopodium*, *Sulphur*, *Calcarea carbonica*, or one of the other polychrests in the first phase. This too makes the choice seem quite difficult.

**The two remedies in the third phase act as *transition* remedies for the particular type of children we are discussing.** *Stramonium* stands between the remedies ruled by the new brain and the remedies ruled by the old brain. In first and second phase remedies, the new brain, the reasoning brain, keeps everyday life in some kind of balance between the conscious and the unconscious. But, in the lower fourth phase remedies, the unconscious rules, and logic gives way to old-brain passions such as hate, lust and uncontrolled appetites.

Standing at the mid-point, *Stramonium* acts as something of a doorway to the unconscious and to the remedies that are ruled by it. In the many references to the unconscious throughout the text, it may seem that I am representing it negatively, as something bad or evil. This is not my intention nor is it my belief. I do not see the unconscious as a demonic monster, but rather as a thing of nature that is somewhat neutral—much as Carl Jung did in his earlier works. What gives voice and color to that neutral thing is the individual's own particular view of the world around him. For example, the child who laughs like a fiend or acts like a demon is only acting out his internalized view of the world. In these children who need third and fourth phase remedies, the coloring of the world is very strong, so strong that it takes control of them.

# STRAMONIUM

*Baryta carbonica*, on the other hand, acts as a doorway to the dulling of the mind and the remedies noted for that. In these upper fourth phase remedies, the brain's functioning is stilled more and more. *Baryta carbonica* is midway between remedies with normal brain function and remedies with dullness.

These two remedies share many symptoms with the first and second phase remedies. Thus all *Stramonium* and *Baryta carbonica* children will have strong symptoms of the *Medorrhinum* and *Tuberculinum* nosodes and also of the polychrests.

As we have seen, **the fourth phase is broken into two categories of remedies**. Those in the bottom portion of the grid are the ones ruled by their passions. In these you will see jealousy, hatred, and violence of all kinds playing an increasing role. The remedies in the top portion show a tendency to become increasingly dull. As expected, all the remedies in the fourth phase share many symptoms with the remedies that came before them. This means that every *Hyoscyamus* child will show some symptoms of *Stramonium* as well as symptoms of one of the nosodes and of some of the polychrests. The *Helleborus* child will have some symptoms of *Baryta carbonica* and one of the nosodes and some of the polychrests.

Please note that there is a pathway in the model to travel from the top fourth phase to the bottom fourth phase. For example, a child whose primary complaint is dullness may be seen, and the prescription turns out to be an easy *Helleborus*. After taking the remedy, the child's issues change from dullness to violence, and the whole state eventually changes into *Hyoscyamus*. After some time, the state may change again from *Hyoscyamus* into *Stramonium*, but it still follows the map.

How can this Map of Hierarchy help us? These days we see many children who may have strong symptoms of four different remedies—for example *Calcarea carbonica*, *Tuberculinum*, *Stramonium*, and *Veratrum album*. Which do we give? How do we decide which of the strong symptoms to pay attention to? We are often faced with this dilemma.

That's where the application of this theory comes in. *If the symptoms we are seeing in all four of the remedies are of equal intensity, it is important to prescribe the remedy farthest to the right, in the fourth phase. If all four remedies come up clear and strong, then obviously the child has held on to the symptoms that came before, and all four states are there. But we can't give all four remedies at once. So in such cases, using Hering's law, we must prescribe for the most severe state and then observe the direction of cure.*

There is yet another application for this theory. As a child moves from the first phase into the second, third, and eventually the fourth, his whole state may *appear* to be difficult to prescribe for. Since he retains many symptoms from each previous state, we are faced with the question of how to use *all* the symptoms. We cannot simply refer to the old books, using the totality of symptoms; they will not bring us to the correct remedy. Until new books are written in a manner similar to this one, showing for example how *Stramonium* shares symptoms with *Tuberculinum* and *Lycopodium,* we will miss the mark if we hope to prescribe for the whole person in this way. Until those books are written, we will have to prescribe on just a portion of the case. In the meantime, we will have to follow Hahnemann's dictate and prescribe on what is most in need of cure at that time.

To take a ridiculous example, but one that will have a familiar ring to it, what would you give to a child who perspires on his scalp during sleep, has slow dentition, is constipated, craves pasta and bread and soft boiled eggs, and hates his brother so much that he has tried to murder him? Now, the whole case description until the end fits *Calcarea carbonica*, but it's that last bit, the murder part, that does not fit. At this point, wouldn't you disregard the perspiration and the soft boiled eggs and start thinking of other remedies, ones that have that last symptom? After all, what is the main complaint of the child? Do we treat this once placid little *Calcarea carbonica* baby whose symptoms are still there, or do we treat the potential murderer? We must pay attention to the symptoms as they relate to the rest of the case, in direct proportion to each other.

When I first began to study homeopathy, I learned that people have constitutional states, or layers, which develop like an onion, one layer upon another. Of course, some children and adults need only one remedy because they seem to be in only one true layer, but others do eventually need more than one remedy. As I near the end of the second decade of my involvement in homeopathy this is still the prevalent, maybe the only, notion that is being learned regarding layers. But there is a problem that is not being voiced loudly enough. While perhaps half the patients seem to fit this nice, neat description of layers, the other half do not fit it at all! For that other half we have had to invent many new models that fit our observations. The Map of Hierarchy is but one such model.

So then, we need to reconsider what treating the whole person means. If we look at these remedies as evolving toward health or disease, we can see in the above hypothetical case that if we use a fourth phase remedy, we are still treating the whole person, because remedies in the deeper phases contain within them symptoms of remedies from the lesser phases.

The description is not complete, and it may well raise as many questions as it solves, but a fuller description will have to wait for a later time and another book. In the meantime, I wanted to share with other homeopaths what I have learned, in the hope that more children will receive help a little sooner. My wish is that it will help the practicing homeopath to gauge what to do *now* in order to provide that help. I also would like to show why and where *Stramonium* fits into the long term treatment of these children. In my first book I described the first two phases. This book describes phase three—*Stramonium*. The third book describes the bottom portion of phase four.

I would like to stress here that the child does not need to be profoundly affected to need *Stramonium*. Since the imbalance may be slight at first, it may only show itself slightly. It is not essential to have the full state to prescribe the remedy. A child who needed *Tuberculinum*, for example, after a fright may have shifted into *Stramonium,* with the case staying much the same as before except for the addition of a few symptoms of *Stramonium* and the disappearance of a few *Tuberculinum* symptoms.

One final word before we look at the *Stramonium* cycle. If you have to make a choice between, let us say, a phase one remedy and a phase four remedy, what will happen if you give the phase one remedy first? Or even a phase two remedy? Should that pose any problem?

Simply put, you must treat the fullest layer that is present at the time. Take an example from my first book. You may see a *Lycopodium* child with arthritis. While the real layer is *Lycopodium,* you may incorrectly assess that the arthritis fits a *Rhus toxicodendron* layer. It would be a mistake to give the latter, because the *Lycopodium* layer encompasses the very symptoms

## THE MAP OF HIERARCHY

that seem to point to *Rhus toxicodendron*. You have to treat the total layer that is on top. There are times when you will see a child who at one point in his life needed a certain remedy but no longer needs it. Now he needs a different remedy. If you give that earlier remedy, the prescription will be incorrect.

There can be serious consequences in some cases. What if you give a remedy that was needed earlier (a healthier remedy or a remedy of an earlier phase) to someone who now needs a later phase remedy? By giving the earlier phase remedy you get rid of some of the symptoms but fail to address the more serious symptoms. These stories should sound very, very familiar to anyone who is practicing, as they occur commonly. One way to put it is to say that the phase one remedy is aimed more at the physical generals, keynotes, and emotional symptoms, and by giving it you get rid of those symptoms and leave behind, in a clearer way, the symptoms of the phase four remedy. So the colds and coryzas and bronchitis are gone and what is left? Intense anger and fear and violence, all of which seem now to be more exaggerated and thus easier to see. This happened because, by giving the remedy underneath, the least severe symptoms are diminished and the most severe symptoms have become more prominent. Traditionally this is called a classic suppression.

There is, however, a second possibility. For a while the remedy you gave seems to be doing a good job on the symptoms you prescribed upon, but the more serious symptoms are still the same. For example, you give *Sulphur* and the child really needed *Stramonium* but you did not see it. Now the *Sulphur* symptoms are better and the child seems healthier in general, but the more severe symptoms (the *Stramonium* symptoms) persist. Now you are stuck with a patient who is clearly better but not well. And eventually these symptoms grow worse. Therefore, we must be very careful in choosing which symptoms to focus upon.

*All symptoms are not equal.* We have to find clear and effective ways to treat what needs to be treated. Whenever we are faced with a difficult choice between remedies, hopefully this knowledge will help us to focus on the most dramatic layer present, the most severe, the most limiting, and thus lead us to find the center of the patient's difficulties. If we can do that, it will then be easier to trace where they came from and see where they are going.

# STRAMONIUM

As mentioned earlier, this whole discussion is expanded upon in the third book. It is presented here to show why the first book contained the remedies it did, why *Stramonium* needs its own book, and finally to present a cosmology of remedies, as they relate to each other.

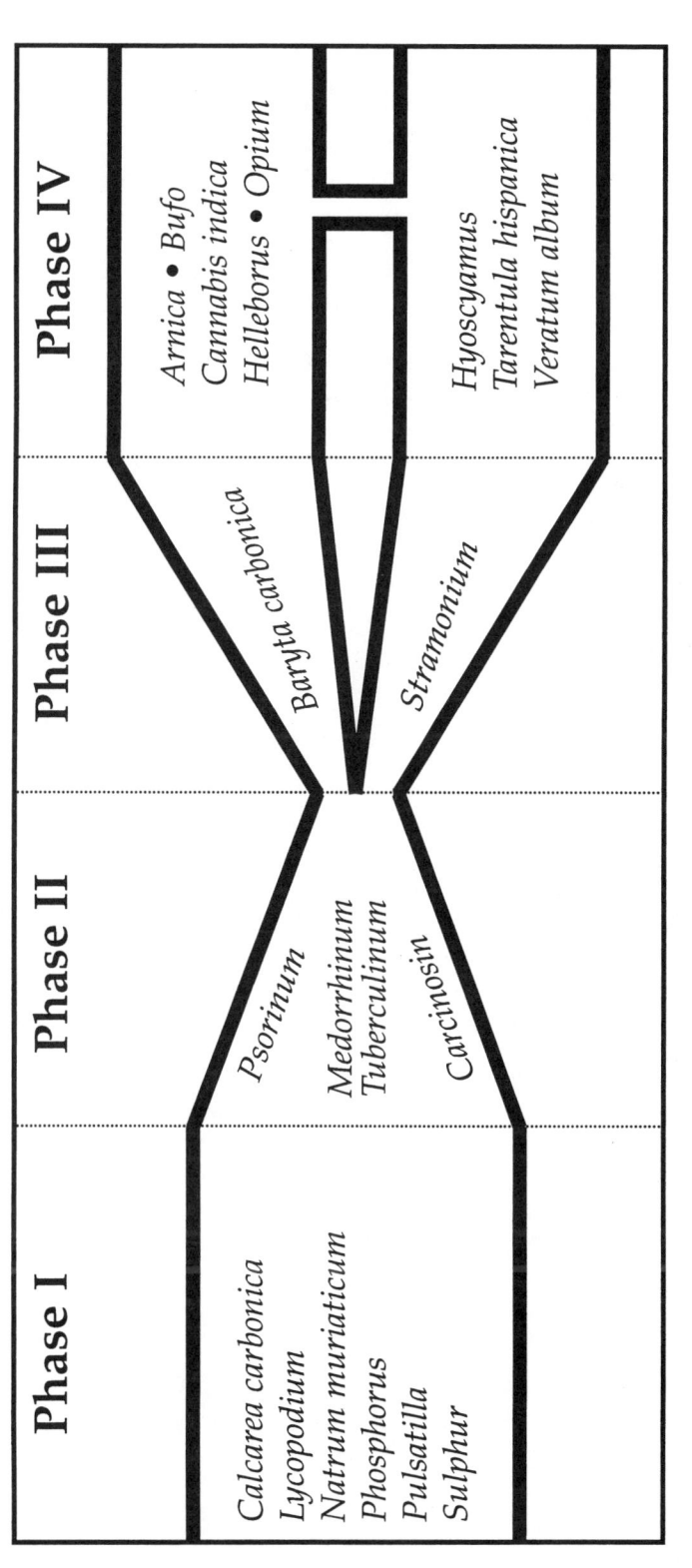

| Phase I | Phase II | Phase III | Phase IV |
|---|---|---|---|
| Calcarea carbonica<br>Lycopodium<br>Natrum muriaticum<br>Phosphorus<br>Pulsatilla<br>Sulphur | Psorinum<br>Medorrhinum<br>Tuberculinum<br>Carcinosin | Baryta carbonica<br>Stramonium | Arnica • Bufo<br>Cannabis indica<br>Helleborus • Opium<br>Hyoscyamus<br>Tarentula hispanica<br>Veratum album |

## The Map of Hierarchy

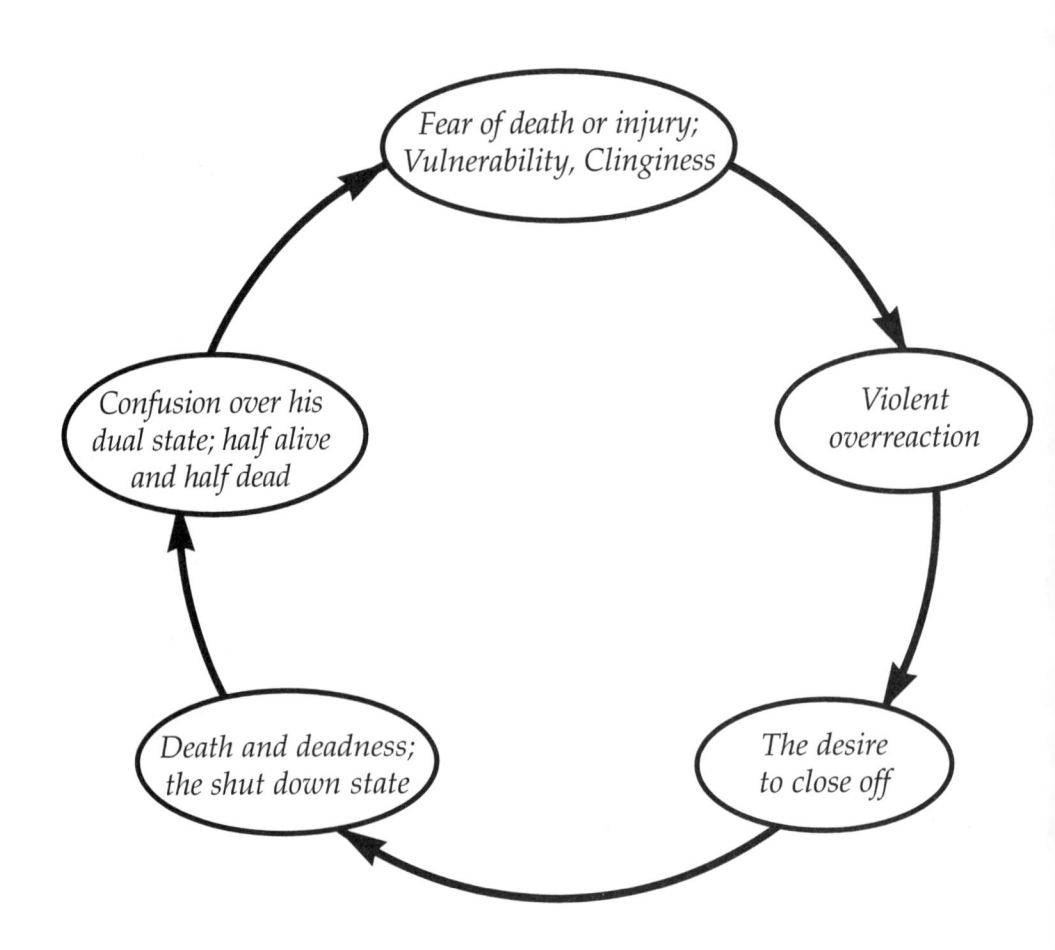

```
                    Fear of death or injury;
                    Vulnerability, Clinginess


  Confusion over his                              Violent
  dual state; half alive                        overreaction
  and half dead


      Death and deadness;                    The desire
       the shut down state                   to close off
```

# The Stramonium Cycle

# *The Stramonium Cycle*

As can be seen in the cycle diagram, the *Stramonium* child is very fearful, he feels alone and vulnerable and thinks that he is going to be hurt. These fears drive him to act, but his actions overshoot, producing unintended consequences—he overreacts in a violent way. Having overreacted, he now has less energy and wants to close off to protect himself and his remaining energies. But again he overshoots and closes off *too* much, so that parts of him become numb, parts of him feel dead. Now images of death, feelings of deadness, and feelings of being alone come up and confuse his experience of reality. The child's overall view of the world is warped, in that everything he experiences goes through this filter of confusion which leads him again to more fear, self protection, overshooting, and then to becoming closed off again.

These children may come to us at any level of pathology, but the more pathological they become, the deeper they travel into the cycle. Some children may only experience this state to a lesser degree, although if they remain untreated they will worsen and fall into a downward spiral until they embody the entire state. Being able to recognize the pattern of this cycle allows us to treat not only these children but also those who have not yet become so terribly imbalanced. We owe it to our patients to know the remedies at each of their stages so that we can see the cycle of pathology before it has a strong hold on the patient. Then we can use homeopathy more effectively as preventive medicine.

All the things that occur in this *Stramonium* cycle fall into place and create the symptoms you will read about in more detail in the materia medica. But I chose to lay out the schema of the cycle at the beginning of the book so that as you learn about each symptom, you can see how it fits into the cycle of this remedy in a predictable and understandable fashion. Like any good tool, it should enable you to expand on the materia medica as you discover other symptoms in your patients that also fit into this cycle, even though they may differ in their specifics. There is a universality to this way of understanding a remedy which is broad enough to absorb all observations about *Stramonium*.

Further, by understanding the underlying pattern of symptoms and how they flow one to the next, your ability to recognize which patients need this remedy will hopefully be greatly enhanced. Please refer back to the cycle often. Use it as the framework for categorizing, remembering and broadening your knowledge of *Stramonium*. If there is a particular segment of this cycle which does not seem clear to you, skip over it and come back after reading about the other fundamental segments or the materia medica. Some people find it easier to start with a linear approach of cause and effect and fill it out later. For many of you it will be a good chapter to return to for review, reinforcement and closure once you have finished the book.

I would like to begin the *Stramonium* cycle by describing each of the five fundamental segments and then portraying the cycle that the segments create. Although it is possible to start with any of the five fundamental segments, I have chosen the **Fears** segment to begin with, since it is one of the best known for the remedy.

## Fear of death or injury; Vulnerability, Clinginess

The *Stramonium* child is sensitive to the outside world, seeing images of death everywhere. This segment represents his first reaction to those images—to be filled with fears which revolve around death and dying. He is terrified of death and terrified of the images of death. His feeling of profound aloneness in this segment is experienced as vulnerability and it is this vulnerability that creates in him a fear of being injured. As you read the first chapter in the materia medica, you will see the many fears that can manifest. Each of those fears is an example of this same issue.

The two segments that lead into this one move the child toward issues of deadness and from there into a state of confusion. This segment shows the first response the child has to that confusion—terror. This terrified state drives him into action. He needs protection and wants protection and will do whatever it takes to get it. That is why he clings desperately to others and tries so hard to communicate. It is also the reason he might try to get out of the situation, to escape. However, in *Stramonium,* his reaction to the fear (the drive for protection) keys up his nervous system and spills into a violent overreaction, which is the next segment of the cycle.

## Violent overreaction

By violent overreaction I mean that the child is propelled into action by the feelings of extreme terror described in the previous segment. It is those fears and the desire to protect himself against them which cause the child to overreact, thus overshooting the intended mark.

This overshooting is a classic problem in systems dynamics and is often found in chronic disease. The vital force creates some structure to save itself and produce a healing result. Instead, the child tries too hard and overshoots his mark, thereby going past where he wanted to end up. Now there is a further imbalance to deal with. The very desire to help himself leads to overshooting and lands him in the violent overreaction segment of the cycle. It is this flaw in the defense mechanism which leads to chronic disease in the first place.

To demonstrate overshooting, let's take a common example, a child who feels abandoned. Either consciously or unconsciously he may try to alleviate this feeling by doing things which will guarantee that he will not be left alone. However, in his panic to attain security he overshoots and becomes extremely clingy, demanding and obnoxious. His needs are so overwhelming that the parents can never give him enough appreciation and so he feels abandoned again. Or even worse, his extreme behavior may drive his loved ones away and then he truly *is* abandoned. This pattern seems to be built into the system.

Let's look at another way that violent overreaction can show itself. Suppose the child is stuck in some situation and frightened. It is natural to seek comfort, but in his eagerness to get it, the nervous system overshoots and the outcome can be anything from stammering or intense blinking to chorea, spasms or seizures. Even the organs have their own way of overreacting, through excessive discharges, excessive urination, diarrhea, or profuse perspiration.

One of the most prominent places affected by violent overreaction is the nervous system. There is one segment of the child that is dead, lifeless, not wishing to live, and so not moving. There is another segment that really is *scared* of death—that wants to live and in so doing wants to move, to communicate, to act. As these two sides keep vying for control of the individual, the battlefield grows larger, affecting more parts of him. The two sides are locked in a tug of war between wanting to move and not wanting to move. Therefore, the nervous system is getting mixed messages and eventually this leads to the spasms, cramping and seizures so often seen in this remedy.

Violent overreaction is also apparent in a type of hypervigilance. On the emotional plane, some children may overreact to a real or imagined hurt by striking, tearing, hitting, and at times actually doing real damage to a person or to property. As these passions are released, the child may begin to actually enjoy violence for violence's sake. These children can even overreact to a bright light or a harsh noise. Sometimes just seeing shiny glittering objects can bring about symptoms such as convulsions. Parts two and three of this materia medica offer many examples of violent reactions or violent acting out.

To summarize, I believe that violent overreactions come out of the fear the child experiences due to feeling alone and unprotected and therefore vulnerable. This leads him to try to reach out, to communicate with others in order to receive their protection and love. But in the rush for that nurturance, in the rush to get emotional needs met, he overshoots the mark and goes beyond what is good for him and those around him into a violent overreaction. It is the most excessive reaction that you will find in the *Stramonium* cycle.

## The desire to close off; Exhaustion

This segment represents the *Stramonium* individual's initial desire to close off, to contain himself. It can develop for different reasons. The child may make a conscious, deliberate choice to try to contain the frightening intensity of the violent overreactions which preceded it. This often manifests as a desire to retreat, as can be seen in the way these patients burrow into their blankets at night, completely covering up. They may push others away, rejecting physical contact.

The other reason for a person closing off may be to conserve energy because he is exhausted. This type of exhaustion and weakness occurs after a great deal of energy has been expended. A good example is the weakness that follows seizures. This closing off segment often contains depression as well, a kind of post adrenal depression in a person who is spent, tired, and failing.

## Death and deadness—the shut down stage

This segment contains a proliferation of symptoms relating to death and deadness in one form or another. It might show up in the eyes as vision loss or sometimes even total blindness. A person's breathing may stop. He might not be able to urinate or defecate. In fact, any element of deadness that a body part can experience, such as a stopped up nose, loss of smell, or numbness of a limb, can take place in this segment. The patient might shut himself down so much that he may even say it feels as if a part of him *is* dead. Other forms of deadness seen here are painlessness of complaints which normally cause pain, and lack of feeling that can follow injury. Autism is an even deeper expression of being shut down, a deadened type of non-communication and non-existence.

It is here in this segment that you find symptoms and symbols of death, such as blackness, coldness, devils, and ghosts. Here the unconscious reigns, conjuring up these images. This segment is the low point in the *Stramonium* cycle, as shut down and contracted as you can become.

When we see all these leanings toward images of death, we have to ask why they exist. Where do they come from? The shut down feelings come from an *overshooting* of the desire to close off, described in the previous segment. The child overshoots to the point of being *too* closed off, so that parts of him actually *feel* dead. This is when the symptoms of deadness of part of him can arise.

## Confusion over his dual state; Confusion about reality, life, and death; issues of being half alive and half dead

This segment deals with the deep confusion existing within the child. It grows out of a dual nature. One side of him wants to live, to thrive and to connect, but instead it overshoots into a violent overreaction. The other side feels too intensely and so he wants to contain that feeling, control it and shut it down. But once again he overshoots and shuts down so much that, in a way, it kills a part of him, producing images, feelings, thoughts and confusion concerning death. And there this child is, the poor *Stramonium*, stuck in a battle between life and death.

This dual nature can be seen in many symptoms of the child: the feeling as if one side is alive and one side dead, as if the body is divided, as if he had two minds. Also found are qualities of indecision and capriciousness. Confusion can be seen as well in the mania symptoms of *Stramonium*. He does not recognize himself, his parents, or other people, seeing them instead as animals or some other thing or being. Night terrors fit in here too, since the child is divided between the waking and sleeping state. In general, there is confusion about what is real and what is unreal. But more specifically the child is confused about his own personal state within that reality.

Where does all this confusion come from? From the fact that one part of him is alive and wants to stay that way and one side of him is dead. That's pretty confusing and upsetting. This confusion follows the segment of images and issues of death and deadness, the shut down state, which eventually flows into the multitude of fears and his desire to do something to stay alive. This creates the dual state, exemplified by the confusion from trying to contain both sides at the same time. And so the cycle is complete, only to start all over again.

## The Cycle

**This then is the cycle: Driven by confusion, fears, and vulnerability, *Stramonium* is engaged in an ongoing and violent battle between the unconscious and the conscious, between darkness and light, between succumbing to the death realm and yearning to exist in the life realm.**

A child feels divided between the conscious mind and the unconscious mind, between life and death, light and darkness. The battle goes on, but there are no clear winners. A precarious balance is established between the part that wants to live and the part that wants to die. But this balance is threatened whenever the child is assaulted by frightening situations or even by images conjured up by his own unconscious mind. With every assault he becomes more fearful, fearful of anything that might disturb the balance, fearful that the dead side will overtake him. So he desperately has to do something about it, such as seeking comfort from loved ones

# THE STRAMONIUM CYCLE

who can pull him out of the dead side and save him, because he knows he cannot win this battle alone. At this point, he is so desperate that the smallest stimulus can trigger a violent response, an overreaction, which comes from trying to stave off the shock and keep away anything that might let the dark side win.

Such a violent outpouring can use up all of his energy, and the intensity of that may frighten his conscious side. Either way, what he ends up doing is beginning to close off, either in order to conserve energy or because the intensity of the violence was too much to bear and he could not understand what was happening.

This closing off then overshoots and continues until the shut down state becomes so severe that he ends up killing off parts of himself. And in doing that he is back to where he began. Now an even bigger part of him is dead. This only serves to deepen the fight between the living and dead sides of him, and then around the cycle he goes again, each time with the symptoms worsening.

For example, after a scary event, the child's fear may produce in him an urgent desire to cling, to communicate. He cannot help himself, so he rushes to express his needs, but instead the nervous system reacts so violently to the ongoing struggle that he can only stand there and stammer. He tries so hard, but the battle rages until he finally succumbs to exhaustion and begins to shy away from even attempting to communicate. At that point he becomes more reclusive, which again brings on the feelings of aloneness, fear, abandonment, and the desire to cling to someone. In this way, the cycle keeps repeating.

And so the child is stuck in this unending cycle—alone and wanting to live, yearning for comfort and nurturing, but each time he reaches for it he overshoots and is misunderstood, and so he winds up becoming even more reclusive and filled more and more with ideas of death. These two sides fight it out every day of the child's life. Every time he tries to get comfort, he unwittingly produces a situation that will push others away and drive him deeper into himself. This is one reason why we find *Stramonium* as a major remedy for the feeling of abandonment and feeling alone in the world. These issues of life and death and the presentiment of death, of fearing death and wanting to live, become the most active poles in the child's life, and a great deal of this book is concerned with these opposing issues.

## A Seesaw War

The nature of the cycle of *Stramonium* is the interaction between two major sides. The unconscious reaches through a gap into the conscious, and the conscious responds, but its response leads it back down the path to the unconscious again. The conscious and the unconscious. When one goes up the other goes down. Up into the world of light and life. Down into the world of darkness and death. This constant struggle produces a lot of the symptoms of *Stramonium*.

*It is the intermingling of the two sides going in opposite directions that gives many of the interesting keynotes pointing to Stramonium.* For instance, convulsions with consciousness, or night terrors in which they seem totally awake, or the delusion that they are half buried, half dead and half alive. That one point is *Stramonium*. The two sides fight it out, one totally alive and fighting to live, and the other dead, wanting to die, and embracing the idea of deadness.

## The Straits of *Stramonium*

So we can see why *Stramonium* is at the crossroads on the Map of Hierarchy—because it seems to rip open the border between the unconscious and the conscious, between the new brain (the cortex) and the old brain (the hypothalamus and limbic system). By tearing asunder the barrier that we all have, the barrier that keeps us 'civilized', it unleashes the passions that we have kept nicely under control and allows our more animal nature to arise and take over, bringing all our emotions to the fore, especially those involving violence and/or fear. Once you have observed these children and seen their violence and fear acted out, you come to truly appreciate how fortunate we are to have been given the gift of reason over passion. These children, lacking that ability, experience terrible suffering.

*Stramonium* stands on the crossroads. Like the phase one remedies, it has the desire to live and to love life, and yet the other side is spiritually unable to support the life process. And that is the essential difference between phases one and four. It is these two issues that *Stramonium* must address. The two issues narrow while passing through the straits of

## THE STRAMONIUM CYCLE

*Stramonium*. In phases one and two, the conscious mind more or less has control of the person, and most of the symptoms listed there easily point to the remedy needed. Thus you can pick just about any symptom of a patient who needs a phase one or two remedy and you'll find the remedy. The lower section of phase four, on the other hand, is all about passions and the old brain. Here the unconscious reigns supreme, unchecked by the conscious side. The most violent of remedies will be found in this phase. The most heinous crimes are committed by people who need remedies in the fourth phase. In the past when we saw these intense symptoms we were obliged to focus on only the most severe part of the case. As we begin to understand the cycles of these remedies and their fundamental segments, we can now look at the totality of the case.

This cycle theory will hopefully give you a better understanding of the how and why of *Stramonium*. Just one word of warning. Not every patient needing *Stramonium* will seem to exhibit all of its symptoms. Some will only have a portion of them and others may seem to only have one. The latter will be the hardest ones to detect. They will not seem to fit the *Stramonium* picture. But if you look deeper you will see it. In every patient needing *Stramonium*, you can count on seeing that intermingling of the conscious and the unconscious, of the life side and the death side.

What is more, careful case taking will show you the whole cycle in every *Stramonium* patient, even if there are things they are not telling you. Close observation of their expression and body language, or sometimes simply the feeling you have in their presence, reveals more than words ever can. If you rely too much on words, the segments may be harder to find. That is, if you are exploring the segment of violence and overreaction, you need not necessarily see *emotional* or intentional violence in the child, but you will see some type of violence somewhere in the case, be it in the violent diarrhea or a violent outpouring of the nervous system, such as in epilepsy.

One last point. Like any cycle, a remedy cycle can be simplified and contracted down to the fewest number of segments possible. Or you can expand the cycle by breaking each segment into several subsegments. Doing that may help you to differentiate this remedy from others like it.

# A Whole Book on Stramonium?

Before 1986 I hardly ever gave *Stramonium*, and when I did it was based upon the rather dramatic symptoms found in the old books. But that year, at a conference, my wife Amy Rothenberg and I heard George Vithoulkas give an excellent one hour presentation that shifted forever my understanding of the remedy. What a shock. He brought this remedy to life in a totally new way, a way that went well beyond what I had previously understood. For the first time I could see how someone who was not maniacal could need *Stramonium*.

Over the next two years it was Amy who prescribed it more times effectively, and I learned much about it from her. It has been my great fortune to be married to such an excellent homeopath—learning has never been far from home. Mulling over what I learned from her, from colleagues, from my own experiences, and from trial and error, I came to see *Stramonium* as an encompassing remedy—one that, like a chameleon, could appear camouflaged as either a polychrest or nosode or as one of the mania remedies. A perfect set-up for confusion and incorrect prescribing.

It is true that the old masters gave us good information about *Stramonium* insofar as it related to delusions, mania and insanity, and that information has been invaluable over the years in helping people who fit those descriptions. However, it no longer seems to be as relevant, for in today's population it is rare to see that type of behavior. Largely due to the extensive use of psychiatric medications, the patients we see now do not usually show the intensity of those extreme symptoms.

But maybe I should stop right now and answer the question that must be on your mind, "Why a whole book on one remedy?" There are a number of reasons.

First of all, *Stramonium* stands at the crossroads, sharing many symptoms with the remedies that come before and after it on the Map of Hierarchy. It is the quintessential remedy for a class of remedies that are regularly used for violent or autistic behavior. A clear and complete picture of

# STRAMONIUM

*Stramonium* is needed because too many of these troubled children will at some point develop symptoms that point either to *Stramonium* or to some remedy that is very similar. Knowing the difference is crucial if we want to help them. This book is a model for how you can view and understand every one of those remedies. If you can see the complete cycle of *Stramonium*, and if you can see how the symptoms group themselves perfectly under the fundamental segments of the cycle, then you can do the same thing for any remedy.

In addition, if you can see how much more serious is the pathology of *Stramonium* than that of the polychrests or nosodes, you will have an easier time understanding the stark intensity of the phase three and four remedies and thus be better able to match remedies to the level of illness in your patients.

Another reason for giving this remedy so much attention is that it is all too often underprescribed because it is easily confused with the polychrests and the nosodes, due to having so many symptoms in common with them. Thus many children who have needed *Stramonium* have gotten the wrong remedy originally and then have been lost in the follow-up.

Oddly enough, it has also been overprescribed, but for a different reason. Because many homeopaths so strongly and correctly associate violence and fear with *Stramonium*, they tend to give it whenever they see such symptoms, without realizing that *Stramonium* is only one remedy from that group and that those symptoms also apply to other phase four remedies.

Another valid reason for painting a fuller picture of *Stramonium* is that many of its physical symptoms are not well known by the homeopathic community, and so all too often when a *Stramonium* patient who is doing well comes down with a cough or some other acute illness, the practitioner changes to a different remedy, not realizing that most of the time simply repeating *Stramonium* would have sufficed, as it still fit the manifesting symptoms.

Maybe I should have listed this reason first, since it is so important. There is a growing *epidemic* of children who need this remedy, probably because of increasingly graphic descriptions of terror and violence promoted by our media culture. They are exposed to these at a very young age via movies, television, videos, games, science fiction horror books, and other

# THE STRAMONIUM CYCLE

frightening things. It is no wonder that those who might by nature be susceptible to this remedy have a greater chance of falling into the *Stramonium* state.

It is unfathomable to many of us why parents would expose tiny children to senseless and overt violence and terror, but expose them, they do. This is a very vulnerable period in children's lives, a time when they are just realizing their individuality and their separateness from their parents. Further, they have not yet learned to discriminate well between fantasy and reality, so when they see violent and scary things, they often think of them as real and that becomes a stress for them, a stress which can result in a *Stramonium* state. Of course, as a child matures, the likelihood of such a response lessens somewhat, but for most children it does remain to some extent for years to come.

In addition to the children who are damaged by this media bombardment, there are those unfortunates who witness violence and horror in their own lives. We are also seeing more *Stramonium* adolescents these days because an increasing number of them are smoking the herb form of this plant to get a cheap and free hallucinogenic effect from it. In so doing, they prove the remedy, usually its darker and more violent aspects.

Moreover, a whole book was needed on *Stramonium* to show how a 'mid-sized' remedy that is partially but not thoroughly known can be expanded and explored. Then, as it is prescribed and its action is observed over time, it will come to be understood as fully as any large polychrest remedy.

Finally, if we hope to understand a remedy, we must understand all of its symptoms, the common and the peculiar, and particularly the symptoms that seem to contradict each other. For example, why do some children who need *Stramonium* love violence and relish horror movies, while others hate them and are afraid of them? We will be better able to answer questions like this once we have understood how opposite ideas can show up in different segments of the remedy cycle, one dominating at one time and the other dominating at another time. What's more, some patients will lean toward one of those opposites, while some patients will favor the other. These nuances are easier to see if the pattern or cycle of the remedy is known.

## STRAMONIUM

After my first book came out, remedies like *Medorrhinum* and *Tuberculinum* began to be prescribed more often because they were better understood for children. I hope that with this book the same thing will happen for *Stramonium*. And as you might guess, I plan to take a very small remedy in a future book and show how that too has a full materia medica associated with it, a materia medica that explains why the symptoms exist in the first place and what patterns you can expect the patient to follow.

Earlier I told you how one lecture changed forever my understanding of *Stramonium*. I hope that this book will do the same for you.

I hope very much that this work will help shed light on the treatment of troubled children. Too many children and too many parents are suffering; may this book help to alleviate some of that suffering.

*\*\*\**

I turn to William James for my closing words:

> "There is but one unconditional commandment, which is that we should seek incessantly, with fear and trembling, so to vote and to act as to bring about the very largest total universe of good which we can see."

# Part Two

## The Materia Medica of *Stramonium*

- Mind
  - Fear
  - Violence
  - Attention Difficulties
  - Introversion
  - Autism
- Sleep
- Body

# *The Element of Fear*

The *Stramonium* child can be consumed by many fears. Before examining these more closely, I would like to emphasize that *all Stramonium fears* (both the familiar ones as well as those highlighted here for the first time) are unleashed by powerful triggers that reflect issues and images of death and of the unconscious. **It is not the specific object of fear that is important, nor even the situation itself. What matters is the *effect* on the child. That is what we need to recognize and that is where we must put our focus. No matter what the stimuli—the effect will be the hideous side of the unconscious ripping through to the side which is desperately trying to create safety, the conscious side. It is this dynamic that makes for a *Stramonium* prescription.** Once this point is understood, it will be easier to see why so many different circumstances can trigger the specific fears of these children, and why it forms the backbone of one of the fundamental segments for this remedy.

It is not fear alone that you are likely to find bursting through, but fear combined with violence. *It is the combination of these two that makes for the prescription.* *Stramonium* shares with *Lycopodium* and *Medorrhinum* the two opposite poles of aggression and inwardness, but with this difference: In *Lycopodium*, the aggressive side shows up in bossiness and irritability, while the inward side exhibits anxiety, lack of courage, and insecurity. (This is described in more detail in my first book, *The Homeopathic Treatment of Children*.) In *Medorrhinum*, the two poles are at more of an extreme, with the difficulty being more one of modulating the intense free-ranging emotions. There is active aggression on the one hand and extremely painful shyness on the other. In *Stramonium*, the boundaries are even further apart. Extreme violence and delirium are on the one side, while on the other side is a fear that borders on, or surpasses, pure panic.

So, a progression can be seen in these three remedies. For *Lycopodium*, the fear is of other people making fun of them or picking on them. For *Medorrhinum*, the fear is often vague; they sense something but may not be sure what it is that they fear or from whence it came, but they do sense that it is a part of their own negative selves, and it is something they do not like. For *Stramonium*, the fear definitely comes from certain stimuli that mirror their inner turmoil. They become most scared of the things that they themselves turn into. For example, the *Stramonium* child who is violent will often fear people and situations that in some way mimic that same violence. It was after such observations that I began to develop the idea of cycles and of these opposite sides within the child, existing together to make up what we know as *Stramonium*. The one side, the side going toward evil and death, is the side that acts out violently. But there is the other side, a side that has a fear of death and the dark, and wants very much to live and to be comforted. That side is being mutilated by the other side.

I think the fears arise in the child because, consciously or unconsciously, he knows the evil that can occur—he knows it personally because he has that death issue, the dark side, within him. He can even reach the point where the unconscious violent side becomes the only filter through which he experiences the world. In that state, he thinks the whole world is just like the horror inside of him, and feeling surrounded by nothing but horror, it is not surprising that so many fears arise.

One of the most consistently seen aspects of *Stramonium* is that the child is living in a perpetual state of fear. After all, if someone's psyche is divided into two sides, one wanting to shut down, eventually hating life and living things and wanting to live in the underworld, and another that wants to live, to grow, and to connect to other living beings—the coexistence of these two will lead to fear. Why? Because of the tug of war between the two sides. The side that desires to live can never be truly innocent since the dark side within his psyche keeps him acutely aware of all the things that can hurt him, all the things that remind him of that dark side, all the things that weaken him and make him drop his guard, thus allowing that other side to take over. He is like a prisoner who has just escaped from his torturer and must keep his wits about him until he is completely safe. Behind every shadow he will see danger lurking. It is never very far—for he carries it within himself. Thus he must be perpetually on guard. Like the terrified being described by Dante in *The Divine Comedy*,"*...as he, who with laboring breath has escaped from the deep to the shore, turns to the perilous waters and gazes...*" so too is *Stramonium* ever fearfully gazing back toward the depths of that unconscious from which he has only temporarily escaped.

# THE ELEMENT OF FEAR

In such a state, it is not surprising that a chronic low-level fear state may, at times, erupt into terror. This is the life of *Stramonium*. So some of these children—the ones who have lost the fight—are violent themselves and live in a violent world and love it. But there are also the children who are paralyzed by their fear; they feel so much terror that they cannot move. The majority, however, fall in between, at times losing all hope, at other times feeling totally free of this fear. But then along comes some event, and it triggers such a strong response of uncontrolled fear, such a primitive reaction, that it shows just how near to the surface the dark side really lies.

## Responses to Fear

The emotional realm of *Stramonium* contains a number of states, such as fear, autism, introversion, and violence. But it is important to realize that a *Stramonium* child may not be violent, may not be introverted, may not be autistic—these states may simply be *reactions* or *responses* to fear, and as such may only exist as long as the situation lasts, otherwise not playing a significant role in the child's life. For example, an event may come up which suddenly jolts the child temporarily into one of these states, but he will recover with time. In some children, however, fear, violence, autism—any one of these states—may take on a life of its own and grow into a permanent state, to be discussed more fully later.

While some children will favor using just one or two of these fear responses, others may revert to several of them at once as ways to escape or to deal with a frightening situation. Any or all of the following responses might be seen at such times: violence, rage, and screaming; crying and depression; clinging to someone; ritualism, autism, and attempts at escape.

### *Violence*

Violence can be a useful response to fear. The familiar preemptive strike, in which the child shifts into an automatic behavior that shocks all those around him, has a solid rationale behind it—it allows him to not acknowledge the fear. With the type of torture he is inflicting at such times, you might expect to see a gloating, sardonic smile. Instead his demeanor seems to say, "Get away from me or you will die! Beware! You might get me, but boy will you pay for it!" You can distinguish it from other remedy behaviors, because it is not a calculated meanness such as some remedies display, but rather a defensive violence. This behavior highlights the fight part of the 'fight or flight' syndrome.

### *Escape*

Another useful response to fear is flight—to escape from the situation. Sometimes the fight reaction kicks in, while at other times the flight reaction, or escape, seems to be the child's only option. We can see the flight acted out in different ways, the most striking being the child actually running away from you or from the room. A less obvious, less dramatic response is the child simply not wanting to be held; he wants to be put down and to go off by himself. Whichever method of escape the child chooses, the point is that the primary goal of this behavior is to deal with his fear.

### *Clinging*

Instead of escaping, some children choose the opposite behavior. They desire to be with people, especially parents and loved ones—and not just to be with them, but to cling to or be carried by them. Again, what these seemingly opposite behaviors have in common is that both help to dispel fear. Whether a child fears a situation in particular or the world in general, he must consciously or unconsciously choose a method of dealing with it. One way is to get support, to seek help from others in order to bolster one's own defenses. If you gather others to your side, it makes you feel less vulnerable, especially if you fear being alone. In such cases the need for people, even clinging to them, becomes essential.

### *Ritualism/Autism*

Fear can also be allayed by going within oneself. If I cannot control the outside world, what is there that I can control? Me. I have to control myself—my actions, even my beliefs. If I can accomplish this, then I can find some amount of comfort. I can predict the future to some extent. I can exercise some control over this crazy universe. For a child who thinks in this way, ritualistic or obsessive compulsive behavior is not uncommon. Even though these behaviors may disappear whenever life becomes safer and more stable, the child may revert to them again each time a stressful situation arises. It is yet another response to fear within the repertoire of the *Stramonium* child. The section on **Autism** and **Introversion** will describe more fully this 'mask of action' as Jung called it.

## *Depression*

When a child grows more fearful and more guarded he may withdraw more and more, and as he interacts with the world less and less, his understanding of it begins to diminish. As the degeneration continues, he may show signs of depression. Some of these children may not know how to verbalize it or might not even realize that they are depressed. But some will feel it keenly and recognize it. By the time a *Stramonium* child reaches the age of six, he may be able to say that there are times he would like to die.

## Vulnerability

One of the outcomes of having to control this dark side within may be the intensifying of a state of fear, a fear of so many things—fear seems to surround the child and be everywhere. He begins to feel vulnerable in this environment, on guard, as if something horrible is going to happen and he will be injured in some way. And because this dark side so colors his perceptions, he believes the injury is bound to come from evildoers, rather than from some natural occurrence. This can lead to many new behaviors. He may become very fearful of strangers, fleeing from them or simply not wanting to go near them. He may even start hitting his mother or sibling, knowing that it will result in a time-out, and he will then be able to go to his room and be away from everyone.

He may also act out in church or synagogue or in any place where there are a lot of people. You may observe in his face or actions that the child is feeling overwhelmed and frightened by this mass of people and needs to get away, to be removed from the situation. If calm enough, he may ask to leave, but more than likely he will already be in an agitated state, no longer able to say what he wants, and therefore he will choose a behavior he knows will produce the desired outcome—immediate removal. He will yell, throw things, hit, push, do anything that the parent will be forced to deal with at once. Often the mother will try to hush the child.

## STRAMONIUM

This does not work. She may then try to hold him on her lap, which also does not work. He just screams louder and begins to push and pummel her. By now the mother is exasperated and removes the child from the crowd. The fact that she is angry with him, that she is yelling at him, that she will take away his privileges—all make it seem as if the child is losing a lot from this behavior. Indeed, in the long term he is losing, but in the short term he has won, for he attained his objective—to leave the crowd. Being there was too scary for him, so he shifted into automatic, not for a moment considering the repercussions. At the time it was an urgent battle for survival.

The *Stramonium* child may be so afraid of people that by the ripe old age of eight to twelve years he may choose not to leave the house, not to go outside and meet friends, not to be with other children or adults. This reclusive type of behavior may at first glance seem to resemble *Baryta carbonica*, but in *Stramonium* it exists for a totally different reason—a deep fear that these people will inflict real harm on him. In *Baryta carbonica* the issue is not so much fear of harm; it is more one of insecurity and embarrassment. The *Baryta carbonica* child hides mostly because he is emotionally thin-skinned, whereas in the *Stramonium* child, the terror of going outside is so strong that if he is forced to, his body may go rigid and he will start rocking in place and moaning. More will be said about *Baryta carbonica* in the next book.

Yet another remedy, *Arnica montana*, can be confused with *Stramonium* because of its vulnerability and desire to avoid people and contact. But the fear in *Arnica* is that as someone approaches, he may touch a tender or bruised area. Clinically, one sees this mostly following an injury. In *Stramonium*, however, the fear is there long before any injury. They fear that if someone approaches, that person may strike them or torture them or abuse them or pick on them. And so any person who draws near to them is seen as a potential intruder, an attacker who means harm. These children experience pain too keenly, and can even feel touch as pain. And so they fear simple touch as one would fear torture. This is why they fear the approach of people.

Picture for a moment this scene. Into your office walks a child who is afraid of injury and of people injuring him, and he has a history to back up this fear. Now here you are, the benevolent homeopath. But what will

## THE ELEMENT OF FEAR

this child's perception of you be? Another doctor, another torturer who will stick this in my ear and poke that in my arm and shove that in my mouth. He can't forget all the vaccinations and shots and tests his parents subjected him to in order to fix whatever was wrong. Now here you are, another doctor who will torment him. Naturally he resists coming into your consulting room, because he does not want to talk to you or even look at you. Instead, he acts out, not caring whether he breaks anything, or whether he gets spanked or yelled at, or anything really. He sets out to create a kind of sixties civil disobedience scene—it does not matter how the point gets across as long as it gets across. His only purpose is to disrupt or even end the visit, or at the very least be taken from the room by one parent, leaving the other to finish the consultation. Escape in any form is enough of a compensation for whatever punishment may be meted out. Punishment is not an issue—fear of injury is. So, in any situation in which the child feels vulnerable, the constant fear that usually lies dormant will suddenly kick into high gear.

He fears that this stranger will deliver the blow that will injure him, the blow he feels must inevitably come—sooner or later. Because of that dual nature existing in the *Stramonium* individual, the living side has to forever contend with the dark shadowy side that is lurking, waiting to harm him.

Vulnerability can be caused by any intrusion—sudden noises, sudden lights, or sudden motions. All these may bring on an immediate feeling of panic or terror. For example, lightning storms may frighten *Stramonium* children, even adolescents, except those who are the violent type, in which case they may actually delight in them. Sudden noises such as those of a vacuum cleaner may create instant terror, and it sometimes takes a while for them to unwind from it. Also if there is a sudden jarring or unexpected motion of the child's car seat or swing or chair, he may let out a shriek, or a look of panic may come over him and remain much longer than it would for other children in the same situation.

*So the dark side colors the imagination with many shades of gray and black, making the child feel vulnerable, fearful of some awful event.* For example, seeing a chain saw may evoke a picture of hands cut off, or seeing a knife may elicit an image of stabbing or some other act of violence—truly "a nightmarish view of life" as the parents of one six year old put it.

# STRAMONIUM

## Fear of Evil

*While the children's fear of being harmed may often be focused on strangers, it is just as often attributed to some supernatural force that is out to get them. This is because that internal dark side colors their perception of the world and of all stimuli they encounter.* That dark side deals not only in frightening things but also in things that have to do with death, such as ghosts. This fear comes out in many of their reactions: a shadow may be seen as a monster or horrible specter lurking in wait, or the noise of a tree limb brushing against the house may be a vampire that is going to suck their blood, or the howling of the wind will turn into the scary screeching of a witch. These are but a few examples of how that dark filter transforms all stimuli into proof that some evil thing is intent on capturing them.

*By far the most common supernatural fears are of ghosts, monsters, devils, vampires, dark shadowy figures,* or things that are under the bed that will reach out and grab them. Ghost stories heard or watched on television can create a state of fear or accentuate an already existing fear, or bring on nightmares or night terrors. The *Stramonium* child who is functioning in the fear realm and struggling to survive may say he is too frightened to stay in the room during the scary part of a movie. Or he may be transfixed by the scene and not be able to turn off the television because what he is watching is so like the dark side he often sees in his imagination. But later, in his sleep, those images of horror may replay as night terrors.

Such children will be afraid that something eerie is going to get them when they are alone, so they will not go to bed by themselves or even go upstairs or to the bathroom by themselves. Something is always lurking and waiting to get them. While fear of devils and thoughts about devils are more well-known for *Hyoscyamus*, clinically *Stramonium* actually comes up more often for this. Devils in movies, picture books, stories—they think all are out to get them, and this increases their fear.

Witches fall into the same category. *Exposure to witch stories, masked faces, and even the occasional bearded man*—all may bring on terror. It is not unusual to find *Stramonium* children from age three to five who not only fear witches but dream of them, and may even have seizure episodes triggered by seeing or hearing stories about them. They may also talk a lot about death or scenes of torture. All these bring up fear of a demonic retribution just around the corner.

## THE ELEMENT OF FEAR

For instance, six year old Eduardo complained of asthma and eczema. He also had exaggerated fears of dogs, the dark, high places, and people hurting him. Television seemed too real for him and he constantly overreacted. It all began at age three when he took a trip to the wax museum. He totally freaked out upon seeing all the decapitated mannequin heads. It got even worse when he watched the machine that cut off the heads at the neck and then drilled holes to make room for the eyes. This came back to him later as an image of people sticking knives into other people's eyes, and became the fodder for many a nightmare and night terror. Ever since that time he had been obsessed with questions of death. When do we die? Can I come back after I die? Will I be alone when I die? He became quite shy outside the house, but at home he was very intense. After *Stramonium* 200C, the asthma and later the eczema ceased, but much more striking was the degree to which his emotional intensity lessened. He was now able to relax with his parents, and with newly found friends at school. Finally he began socializing easily with schoolmates, and all the fears and obsessions left.

Another child at the age of ten went to Christmas mass and heard that Christ died for him and that his soul would be lost if he did not follow all the rules. He developed an overwhelming fear of death that took over and controlled his life.

Twelve year old Jared complained of both headaches and nightmares. Upon questioning we found that he also had fears *of ghosts, bugs, snakes, thunderstorms, and scary movies—movies with violent people, or movies of snakes. These movies gave him night terrors.* He also had nightmares that his parents were in car crashes. He threw temper tantrums when told to take a bath. He has been afraid of ghosts ever since he went to a museum in Salem, Massachusetts where they talked about the witch hunts. Since then he also fears being alone in the dark and must sleep with the light on, occasionally waking up at night really scared, thinking there are ghosts all around him. He gets up at night and sleepwalks. One time he fell down the stairs. Sometimes at night he will scream, "There's ghosts in my furniture!" He hates to sleep in his room any more, preferring the couch in the living room for the last half year. When I asked him why, he told me that at night he sees these visions of ghosts, "coming to get me. I'm in an old graveyard, and dead people are rising out of the grave half rotten and are coming to get me."

Cemeteries also pose problems for these children. The child's imagination takes off and he begins to see the dead bodies coming out and attacking him. If you can recall feeling frightened while watching a similar scene in the theater, these children not only feel that fear, but may actually see the scene as a real event. In this state, the child may resemble *Argentum nitricum*. The same symptom may be there, but this need not confuse you, for the reasons for it are very different. With *Stramonium* it is not the image that we focus on but the reaction to the image, the eruption of the whole terror side and all that goes with it.

The fears do not always have to be so severe or so frightening as those felt about witches or dogs. A child could also be afraid of some event or thing that most children like, such as masks, children with painted faces, men with beards, a man holding a camera up to his face, or even clowns and puppet shows—any of these may frighten a child so much that he cannot sit through the event. Even benign shows like those shown on public educational television may frighten some children so much that they will not watch them. Once again, it is not the stress itself but rather the visual image that, at that moment, allows the dark side to reign over the introverted, frightened side. This glimpse into the death side increases the confusion between the two sides and the confusion brings up fear.

## Fear with Upper Respiratory Infections

Many times the parents will recall that the fears first developed around the time of an upper respiratory tract infection, or a cough or bronchitis with a fever, or an ear infection or streptococcal infection, or when the child had measles or roseola. If asked, they may even say that their child had experienced some fright a short time before the illness began, and that it seemed as though the infection started after the child had recovered from the fright, and along with it this fearful state appeared. Under these circumstances, the child will undoubtedly want the parent and will ask to be held and protected. The parents find it strange that this child, usually so mischievous and rambunctious, can during a fever suddenly become so calm and quiet and sweet, and even beg to be held. I believe that the fever in some way alters the child's perceptions of the world and that the alteration either brings on a fright or accentuates an already fearful state, either one putting the child into a *Stramonium* state.

## THE ELEMENT OF FEAR

For example, Harriett, who is eight years old, developed a cough. She awoke at midnight with a high fever and was extremely frightened. When asked why, she said that everything looked so big. She was very scared and clung to her mother for dear life. She begged for help, talked too fast, said she needed to go to the hospital, and again said everything was so big. Her father asked her to go to the bathroom to try to urinate and she did, but she ran out and came back shrieking and pointing at the bathroom. She was totally hysterical and looked terrified and confused. After ten minutes she settled down enough to say that she had seen some hairy monster in the toilet bowl. For the next eight days, she woke up with night terrors and coughs at midnight. Ever since, each time she has been ill, she has awakened between midnight and two, frightened and screaming for help. She also developed fears of ghosts, death, and the dark. After receiving *Stramonium* 200C she became less shy, less introverted, less fearful and stopped having her recurring cough.

I think that some altered state of perception in these children leads to fears of people or faces or animals. This would explain why the remedy is so useful in states of delusion in which the person actually sees diabolical faces or evil things. It is as if the altered state that develops during the fever leads right into a delusional *Stramonium* state.

### Fear of Animals

Just as people may be viewed as threatening, animals may seem even more threatening. After all, animals have a certain unpredictability; they live closer to their instincts, as the dark *Stramonium* does. Perhaps, to a certain extent, animals may remind the child of the dark animal side within him which then produces fear. He might also be fearful of what could happen to him if one of those carnivores with huge, sharp teeth were to catch him. But since we are rarely around that type of mammal, the dog serves as his object of fear. However, it does not stop there: *wolves, lions, tigers, bears, cats, snakes, tarantulas, bats, rats, and bugs—all these may frighten him*. And the child's worst fear is that these animals will bite him or tear him to pieces.

*This basic fear of animals is often accentuated if the animal is black.* Black cats and especially black dogs may make the child lose reason completely and run screaming to mother, but by the time she picks him up, he may have already passed through to the violent overreaction segment and be so out of control he will be tearing and clawing at her. Even watching a video or movie of an animal, especially a black one, may make him scream or run out of the room or sit mesmerized, only to have a night terror later. Or, upon seeing a black dog on the street, the child may be unable to move, frozen by terror, and start moaning in a low guttural tone, "Pick me up. Pick me up," as he shakes from fright. The child may even begin to grow overly cautious, not wanting to go outside because some animal might get him.

Of course, the worst situation is one in which the animal in question belongs to a relative. The family goes to visit relatives, and while the child is at their house playing, their black dog decides to join the fun and playfully jumps up on the child. The child completely goes berserk, screaming, running, hitting, falling, going totally out of control. After a while he may calm down, but then later he becomes sick with some infection (such as a streptococcal throat infection) or perhaps starts having nightmares. While any child can react with fright to such an event, the threshold is much lower for the *Stramonium* child: the dog need not be as big, nor jump as high, nor act as wild. For such a child the recovery time will be much longer.

Some children may be so terrified at the prospect of a dog attacking them and may feel so little power to stop that assault, that they may not want to leave the house. After a great deal of psychotherapy and talking about it, perhaps their fears will be somewhat palliated if they can hold on to the parent with one hand and their 'power pack' with the other. In the pack is a spray that can temporarily blind an animal, as well as a whistle that is so painful to a dog's ears that it will not come near. Of course the pack only works if the child is with the parent, because if he is alone, his terror is so great that he is unable to work the zipper on the pack. This leaves him with two alternatives—to scream and run, or to freeze and quake and moan for mommy or daddy.

The fear of animals is often found in combination with other fears. For instance, one boy also has a fear of thunderstorms, being left alone, ghosts, and the dark. In addition, his mother must lie down with him for him to be able to fall asleep. He shrinks in fear from animals of all kinds, even frogs— a fear not known to belong to *Stramonium,* and yet it has been cured by it.

THE ELEMENT OF FEAR

**I would like to again emphasize that what really counts is the *reaction* to the stress, as well as how that stress relates to the *Stramonium* cycle. It is not the specific fear itself that will lead us to the remedy, but finding out why that fear exists in the first place.** As such, it is not surprising that some children needing *Stramonium* will not have the fear of dogs it is so well known for, but may rather have an overwhelming fear of something else such as snakes. Why snakes? Because of the way they come and attack you. As one seven year old put it, "Especially the spitting Cobra. It spits poison into your face from far away."

## Hypervigilance

One of the effects of living in a constant state of fear is that you become hypervigilant. After all, if you feel as though the place you are in is a frightening or threatening place, your senses may become very acute, and you will probably become excessively aware of every single thing around you, as well as of each of your own actions as they relate to others. You will be much more cautious, more careful doing anything or going anywhere. For this reason *caution becomes a large part of the fearful Stramonium individual.* As mentioned earlier, one way that the caution can express itself is through a sense of apprehension if anyone approaches them.

An offshoot of this hypervigilance is becoming so controlling of your own actions that you carry it to extremes. The natural extension of that is to move into a whole new segment, one in which self blame is strong any time you do not measure up to your own harsh expectations. Such a child, thinking he has done something wrong will become morose, and feeling that he is incapable will become depressed and think that maybe—just maybe—he should end it all. This is one of the times that the eight to thirteen year old *Stramonium* may want to kill himself and be done with life. This state, in which anxiety of conscience has overwhelmed the child, can easily be confused with *Natrum muriaticum* or *Staphysagria*. It is a state in which the side that wants to live has tried so hard and has compensated so much and become so overcontrolled that the child gives up the fight and resigns himself to hell—he cannot fight any longer.

Once again we have to ask *why* any symptom exists? Why is there this excessive cautiousness? It is not the cautiousness itself or the fear of

# STRAMONIUM

a black dog or any specific symptom that we should be concerned with, but rather why that symptom exists and how it plays itself out. For example, you may see a teenager who goes rigid with fright on ladders or balconies or in trees or any high place. You may be already thinking of *Stramonium* for this young man but cannot find it listed under the fear of heights rubrics in the repertory. You may not even find it in the materia medica. But if you ask him why he has that fear, his answer may be something like, "I'm afraid I'll fall and die." And there is your *Stramonium*, with its fear of death and all the things surrounding death. So it is not the symptoms but the reason behind it that should be our focus when we are talking with the patient.

## Fear in Infants

*Stramonium* is a remedy that can be needed from the very first moment of life. Therefore it is fitting to include a section on the fears of *Stramonium* infants. What we often find is that the birth process itself, in the predisposed child, can push the infant into a *Stramonium* state. He is afraid of: the dark (the womb) and the light (coming out into a too brightly lit world), confined spaces (passing through the birth canal) and being abandoned (wanting to be held as we were at birth). We know these opposing fears exist in the baby, because he may cry hysterically in the dark as well as in bright light, and when he is not held as well as when he is swaddled too tightly.

Thus the fears show such contradictions: aversion to dark as well as light, and aversion to being held countered by the desire to be held. Due to the paradoxical nature of these fears, the parents may at first find it difficult to understand what is wrong. They think the child has colic or an ear infection or such, but over time they simply become exhausted from the constant screaming and the sleepless nights and begin to conclude that they just have a difficult baby. One of the greatest benefits of recognizing this aspect of *Stramonium* is that you can then explain to the parents what their preverbal infant is probably experiencing, and they, in turn, can create a better environment, one that is less threatening to the child. I have seen a difficult situation of this kind completely reversed within four days, given the proper treatment. After the remedy the infant suddenly stops crying and begins to smile and enjoy life more.

# THE ELEMENT OF FEAR

Let us examine some of the fears of *Stramonium* in closer detail.

## Fear of the Dark

*One important Stramonium keynote that is consistently seen is fear of the dark.* When it is found, it is almost always a prominent part of the case. The night terrors that the child experiences are described more fully in the *Sleep* section, as are some of the behaviors of the children at night in the dark, but it is worth mentioning a few of them here. Later when these children become teenagers or adults, they may be able to express what they used to feel in the dark as youngsters but couldn't articulate then: *in darkness the world seems chaotic and threatening.* "How can I know what is going on around me in the dark? I need to keep my lights on so I can tell what is real and what isn't." These thoughts give us a glimpse of what the child is afraid of; since anything can happen in the dark, it heightens his already existing fear of injury. The child is being haunted by his unconscious and his imagination. He loses his ability to evaluate what is real and what is imagined (and therefore real to him alone). He loses his clarity regarding the world. "I can't keep my balance." In a sense, the balance the child speaks of is a balance between the two poles of *Stramonium*. In the dark, the fearful side of the child, the side that desires to live, becomes even more fearful and feels hampered or closed in by the dark threatening side of his psyche. **Darkness magnifies the segment having to do with death. That confuses the child, and as the confusion segment grows, it increases the fear segment.**

Again, it is not the fear of the dark itself that is the issue. If you can get these children to say enough about their fear and to express it clearly, what they tell you will fit very nicely the cycle described in the book. It is in the dark that ghosts, monsters and animals appear. And so the fear is not of the dark itself, but of the monsters that come in the dark. "He has a terrible fear of monsters, which seems to be growing stronger as he gets older. He looks under his bed and in closets, and is afraid of his own shadow and the shadows that appear on the walls at night," is a common report from the parents. So, for these kids, *fear of the dark is actually a fear of being hurt by monsters coming at them in the dark.* And the darkness magnifies the images of death which then create fear.

But there are other children for whom fear of the dark is a fear of enclosed spaces. *The dark has a claustrophobic effect* on these children. They feel cornered, hampered, immobile, in the dark. The horror out there is closing in on them.

For yet another type of child, **the dark accentuates the sense of isolation and fear of being alone.** For instance, Angie from Austria is so afraid of the dark that at night she feels panic and begins to scream unless one of her parents is near her or at least within sight. "One way we've gotten around that is by putting on the radio or a cassette tape at bedtime. The sound seems to relax her." So with these children it is not really a fear of the dark but rather a fear of being alone in the dark. The sound of the radio may lessen the fear. The fear is also diminished if the parent sleeps in the same bed with the child, who will do whatever he can to achieve that goal. Sleeping with the parents may even eliminate his need to have the lights on. At this point the homeopath might miss the remedy due to the absence of the keynote of fear of the dark. Upon questioning though, you may find that this fear returns when the parent stops sleeping with the child.

Another thing to note is that *the child will display more fears during the winter months,* when there is more darkness and less sunlight. In the evening, at an hour when it would still be light in summer, the child, still awake, may have the occasion to go outside. Imagine this scene. It is December, 6 p.m., and the family wants to go out for supper. Everyone is dressed and ready, but when the time comes to go out to the car, the *Stramonium* child is not about to budge. You pick him up and carry him to the car, and he starts shrieking and screaming with fright. If you turn on the inside car light, he relaxes a little, enough to tell you he is scared. You try to reassure him. You tell him he is safe, that it is not night, and that it is normal for it to be this dark in wintertime. But he is terrified. He keeps screaming obstinately that he wants to go back into the house. Finally, if you offer to leave the light on in the car, he may settle down. Winter, when the world is darker, is also when nature, sleeping, looks more dead then ever.

Another common scenario in our modern age, one that exemplifies the cycle of the pathology, is a *Stramonium* child on an airplane. At first, the child may be having fun, restlessly jumping around on the seats, but then the loudspeaker goes on and the flight attendant says that the plane is getting ready to taxi down the runway, so everyone must take their seats and buckle their safety belts. Now the parent has to make the child settle down and be buckled in or be held. He does not like that and struggles to get free. The circumstance, however, dictates that the parent must hold on to him, and so the grip gets tighter. By now the child is feeling claustrophobic and fights to escape, perhaps even begins to yell a little. The parent, slightly embarrassed, tells him that he must settle down and be buckled in, but he refuses. Now the airplane is positioned on the runway, the engines get louder, the airplane begins to shake. And wouldn't you know it, just then the lights dim. The *Stramonium* goes manic at this point, thrashing, shrieking, needing to escape, but the harder he fights, the harder the parent has to restrain him, which only exacerbates things.

This is reminiscent of what happens during the night terrors that are described in the *Sleep* section. Both illustrate how any situation that includes a darkened place as well as being restrained can lead to terror. Thus we can see that it is essential to look beyond a particular symptom in order to see the whole situation in context and thereby understand the complete cycle of the pathology. Once we see this, we will better understand why a particular remedy has a particular symptom in the first place.

Another expression of fear of the dark in *Stramonium* children can be seen in the fear of anything that is a dark color, whether it be dark people, dark animals like panthers, dark basements, dark halls such as movie theaters, or even a dimly lit closet. Playing a trick on a sibling or friend by locking him in the closet has made more than one child into a *Stramonium*.

An interesting offshoot occurred in the case of one child, when the remedy produced a new symptom before completing the cure. This illustrates once again the idea that fear at night can be connected to fear of being hurt. "After the remedy was given, his fears began to slowly fade. But one completely new fear came out. He became scared of bad people hurting him. He would run around the house at night to make sure all the doors were locked. Now he locks the car door, bathroom door, and every door he can find."

*When there is fear of the dark, it will ultimately lead to desire for light, one of Stramonium's more familiar keynotes.* This may be taken quite literally— the child wants to have a light on. Or it can be taken figuratively—children or adults who are seeking some spiritual enlightenment as a way to get them out of the hell they find themselves in. More regarding fear of the dark can be found in the *Sleep* section.

*Oddly enough, because of the cyclical nature of Stramonium, sometimes you may find desire for the dark and fear of light.* This is noted strongly in the remedy. The books describe an intense aversion, on the point of maniacal rage, that crops up when a person sees a brightly lit object. In actuality this extreme form of photophobia is rarely seen. There is, though, the occasional child who, during fever (or other states in which he is delirious, manic, or in the middle of a schizophrenic break) may panic or become violent upon seeing the reflection of sunlight on glass.

At the same time, the fascination that some of these children have with darkness is interesting. Though fearing darkness, they may strangely enough be drawn to it, and actually start to like it more than the light. These are the children that later go on to become fearful of the light; they begin to crave the darkness and feel at one with the night. Usually they are the ones who grow up to become violent or develop autistic traits. These symptoms will be seen in the child who is in the stage of closing off.

## Fear of Being Alone

*High on the list is the fear of being alone.* Though not well known for this symptom, *Stramonium* often has a fear and feeling of abandonment as the root cause of the pathology. That is why the remedy is listed in italics in the rubric, **MIND: Forsaken, feeling** as well as being listed in **MIND: Delusion, deserted.** I have found this issue of abandonment to either be a catalyst that enlarges the *Stramonium* state or simply a feeling many *Stramonium* children and adults have. Whether the child actually was deserted, or whether he just has a feeling of being forsaken—in either case, he acts as if it were real.

The *sense of abandonment* can have its origins in an unwanted pregnancy in which the parents do not try to bond to the fetus. Or it can come from complications during labor in which an injury to the mother leaves her incapable of bonding with the infant or caring for it after the birth. Sometimes it can occur when the infant is in some kind of difficulty and has to be isolated from the parents in an incubator. Or abandonment

## THE ELEMENT OF FEAR

issues may begin at some later time, when the child finds that the parent/parents are not around and are not bonding with him, thus leaving him on his own, and, in a sense, abandoned. In cases in which the child has been physically/emotionally/sexually abused by one of the care givers, he can feel forsaken or isolated and often will be frightened to be alone.

It is unfortunate that many of the fears children encounter in our society are experienced when they are not around supporting, loving adults. It is during these alone times that their unconscious arises in them, unleashing the feeling of terror, and they are on their own to deal with it. So often terror and isolation seem to go together, the fear joined to the sense that they are all alone. As one reads of the many fears of *Stramonium*, he will see one recurring theme—these fears are experienced when the child feels isolated.

The fear of being alone is most accentuated under some of the following circumstances: when the child is in the dark, or after being frightened by some eerie movie, or when the child, in pain, surrenders to the pain, becoming almost unaware of the world around him. These situations can bring on the shut down/dead segment, in which he may hide or retreat into a fetal position (to lessen the pain), or he may cling to the mother as if his life depended on it. Some may express it not as a strong fear, but as hating to be alone, or always wanting to be with someone. However, the root is the same—fear.

The significance of all the clinging, wanting to be held, wanting to sleep with the parent, and wanting loved ones around is that all these are reactions, outgrowths of the child's feeling of abandonment combined with fears for his safety. It is interesting to note that if you, as the homeopath, make contact with the child, he may cling to you and tell you anything you wish to know. If that happens, you will no longer be talking to a reticent child but to someone who wants to please you. For instance, six year old Troy and I hit that point in the interview, and from then on all I had to do was ask and he freely volunteered much more, as in the following exchange. I asked Troy what he feared. He reeled off a list: being alone, the dark, storms, scary movies, broken glass, and others. He talked so fast as he answered that he was sucking up air, garbling words, and spitting them out all mixed together.

As mentioned in the description of the cycle and in the *Autism* section, the child can and often does retreat into his own world and seems to live a solitary life. In the various rubrics of delusions that relate to being alone in the world, *Stramonium* is well represented. In such cases it will be the child, not the parent, who severs the bond.

## Claustrophobia

*A fear of closed-in spaces* is not as universal for *Stramonium* as the fears previously mentioned and yet it does fit in with the ideas discussed thus far. Perhaps it would help to list a few rubrics for *Stramonium* that are in the repertory: **MIND: Delusion, buried alive; MIND: Delusion, in his grave; MIND: Delusion, side, alive on one and buried on the other, he is; MIND: Fear, tunnels;** and **MIND: Fear, narrow places.**

From early on, you will see the sense of isolation and abandonment as well as the fear of being enclosed or trapped—all keynotes of the *Stramonium* state. This remedy has also been found to be good for claustrophobic adults who display a fear of narrow places or tunnels. Children too may have this fear. It can be observed at the playground, in the child who will not crawl through the tube. He may likewise refuse to go down a slide, especially a circular slide, especially if the slide is enclosed by a tube, and most especially if there are children at the bottom of the slide making noises that echo up the tube to where the *Stramonium* child stands. Similarly, he may not wish to go into a maze, even if his siblings are going in. It is just too confining and dark for him.

*At night or sometimes even during the day these children may not want doors closed, or may dislike elevators, or may take a very long time to calm down after their siblings have locked them in the bathroom for a few minutes as a gag. They may even start having nightmares as a result.* They may also exhibit a fear of going into closets at all, or not want to play in big empty cartons from refrigerators or other large appliances. These children may not even like hugs or any activity that makes them feel confined, such as being pinned down for a time-out or being tackled in football. And, as mentioned already, the *Stramonium* infant, when swaddled, may struggle from fear of confinement.

Different children express this claustrophobic fear in different ways. One may say he feels trapped or hemmed in by his surroundings. Another may feel suffocated or as if he is being choked. *The materia medica*

# THE ELEMENT OF FEAR

*refers to this state in various ways, but feeling as if you are in a grave or buried alive really captures the feeling—that is the epitome of being trapped in a hostile environment. The fears are only a reaction to this intense feeling*

An opposite tendency to claustrophobia sometimes may be seen in a child who has autistic traits or is in the process of closing down (*i.e.*, the shutting down and the shut down/dead segments). This child may actually prefer being in confined spaces, as this lessens the overstimulation that he feels. Such a child may often be found under the bed, behind the furniture, in the closet, and in other enclosed spaces. Do not be limited in your thinking by assuming that it is only the fear of enclosed spaces that is typical of *Stramonium*, for the remedy actually encompasses both extremes.

## Fear of Water

*Water presents a special problem for the Stramonium child. Many of them will have an intense fear of water, especially of showers or of getting the head wet.* The child needs his hair washed, but getting him into the bath is a totally miserable chore for parent and child alike. "It's a horrible time for all of us." The child struggles as if his very life depends on staying out of that bath. Many a *Stramonium* state has either originated in or been accentuated by forcing a child like this into the shower or bath. I have treated children who, after being coerced, developed nightmares or night terrors or twitches or even seizures.

Worse still is the child who is thrown into a pool or lake to make him learn how to swim. By the time the parent has finally torn away his grip and tossed him into the water, the child is already so terrified that he panics, becomes stiff and rigid, and fights so hard against the water that if the parent did not jump in to rescue him, he would probably drown. If, by luck, the child manages to reach solid ground on his own, the trauma still will have been so severe that the effect on him may be far-reaching and extreme.

What is most striking is to see a tough and violent kid (who lords it over others and is known as the town bully) fall apart at a birthday swimming pool party, where he is afraid to go into anything but the kiddie pool. Or, in the park, where all the other kids run in and out of the fountain, splashing each other, this bully becomes unusually reclusive, sticking near his mother or playing near the fountain but not willing to go in.

# STRAMONIUM

Or perhaps he goes in, but only if he can hold on to his mother. However, if he does release his grip and begin to play, if he finally drops his guard and goes in the water, the moment it is splashed in his eyes, or some child douses everyone by spouting the fountain, it is the *Stramonium* child who will get scared and run out. The rest of the children will be squealing gleefully or hooting in mock protest.

Water may aggravate this kind of child for several reasons. First of all, it is not so much that the water hurts his eyes, but more that it intrudes into his psychic space. It is the intrusion that is the point of sensitivity. Particularly intolerable is an intrusion into the eyes, since the eyes can be considered an extension of the brain (so closely connected that the slightest injury can paralyze him in the moment). The sudden temporary blindness caused by the water frightens the child because his dark side, his unconscious side that so torments him, is victorious for the moment. In addition, this temporary blindness from the water can produce a claustrophobic effect. Since it prevents the child from moving, he feels stuck and is frightened because he does not know what is going to happen to him.

Water may also be thought of metaphorically in relation to *Stramonium*. Jung hypothesizes that water represents the unconscious realm within the person, the fluid aspect, and Melville idealized the relationship between the unconscious and water in Moby Dick, "Let the most absentminded of men be plunged in his deepest reveries—stand that man upon his legs, set his feet a-going, and he will infallibly lead you to water, if water there be in all that region…Meditation and water are wedded forever."

Throwing water into the child's face not only blinds the conscious side, but also adds water to it—that is, expands the unconscious. In the cycle of *Stramonium*, balance depends on the conscious mind remaining vigilant in order to counter the efforts of the unconscious mind to take over. If the conscious mind loses control or is put in a situation where the unconscious erupts, there is the potential of a tilting of the scales. In addition, in order to maintain the balance that the child feels he needs to survive, since water is fluid, he becomes the opposite of fluid—rigid, inflexible, ritualistic. This side cannot allow his guard to drop and so is aggravated by this burst of fluid. I think that this may be what is behind the child's fear of water in general. It has such an intense effect on him that it keeps him from going into the water. Take a five or six year old who has not only the aforementioned fears but also a fear of the ocean—and not just of swimming in the ocean but even of being near it. He may become so terrified by watching the waves ebb and flow and looking out at this huge expanse of water, that his body becomes rigid, and he will scream to be picked up and held and taken away from this horrible scene.

If this theory is correct, then throwing water in the eyes of a child like this, or submerging his head in water, or throwing him into a lake to teach him how to swim is just as terrifying as hurling an image of a devil at him, or leaving him alone in a scary museum, or plunging him into darkness. All these things exaggerate that which is already inside the child, that segment of death, and all of a sudden he feels as if the light side of him is losing. In this respect, the fears of water are very similar to the fears of darkness.

## Ailments from Fright

As was stated in the introduction, I believe that a remedy state actually exists as a stable pattern that may be best viewed as a *systems dynamics* version of an addiction loop. In a loop there is no real beginning or end, and one can enter it from any location on the circle. *One place where it seems that people readily enter the Stramonium loop is via a fright.* I think this is the case with many children, such as a child who fears dogs after being attacked by one, or one who fears closed-in spaces after being locked in a closet by mistake, or even a child who fears sudden sharp noises such as water rushing into the bathtub or the sound of jet airplanes shooting overhead, because when his mother was pregnant with him, she was frightened by a dangerously low flying loud plane. Just as likely, these children may have been in a *Stramonium* state already, but it only became clear when a fright accentuated the symptoms. For example, a child who already has learning difficulties and is slightly physically awkward in gross motor skills, may develop fears, violence, and night terrors after seeing a scary movie, topped off by being left alone.

## Similarity to *Baryta carbonica*

To a certain extent, *Stramonium* with its many fears may present like *Baryta carbonica*. For example, Roger, age five, was afraid of insects, witches, ghosts, thunder, loud noises, the dark, and dogs. He was slow in learning

## STRAMONIUM

to walk and talk, he toilet trained late, and had poor fine motor coordination; in short his evaluation by his developmental team was that Roger was quite emotionally delayed. Because of his inability to interact appropriately, he began withdrawing from the other children. These symptoms, while being more well known for *Baryta carbonica*, are also shared by *Stramonium*. So, what made for the *Stramonium* prescription in this case? There was another side to Roger besides this fearful side; he was contrary, always arguing with others, hitting his parents, refusing commands, and complaining at school. He was also obsessed with the metaphysical, most especially with death and dying, with leaving the body, and with ghosts. The parents had brought him for treatment because he had developed seizures and was about to be put on medication. One dose of *Stramonium* 200C, and later one dose of *Stramonium* 1M, stopped the seizures, as well as the behaviors mentioned. His fears ceased, as did the aggression and the preoccupation with the occult. Instead, he went through a period during which he had upper respiratory tract infections before finally being well.

Then there is Sally, a five year old girl whose chief complaint is fear and nightmares. Her fear is especially of the dark, being alone in the dark, the basement, lions, tigers, and bears, lightning, and thunder. She fears that her mother may die. "My cat died and my mom might too." She worries about people in the family dying from germs. Her mother relates, "She often vomited in her sleep as a baby, and maybe she started being frightened then." She talks to her parents a lot about death. She tells them that she has dreams of nails being driven into her eyes, dreams of monsters and of accidents. She will wake and go into her mother's room. In the interview she seemed sweet and gentle, but when I checked to confirm, her mother said that she is sweet but can be very stubborn as well, cuddly but also complaining. When I asked Sally if she ever hits other kids, she said, "No I just smack them. Smacking hurts a lot more than hitting."

### Contradictions Within the Remedy

As mentioned earlier, I feel that any description of a remedy must in some way try to address disparate symptoms and apparent contradictions within that remedy. How can the same remedy have both a fear of the outside and a fear of being confined? Or how could a little child have a strong fear of some people and yet be biting others? I think the premise of this book (vitalism and the cyclical nature of disease) explains not only why such divergent symptoms can coexist in one person, but also how they operate within the cycle of the disease. A lot of the reactions to fear, though they may seem at first to be contradictory to each other, point to that segment which contains presentiment of death and images of death and of being alone, which lead to a multitude of fears that the child will then have to address.

## After the Remedy

Within weeks to a month after the remedy, the fears will begin to disappear. In the case of Alex, "The fear of water disappeared, making bathtime much easier. No more screaming or fighting." While he still talked about monsters, he no longer cried about it, nor did he have to check under the bed or in the closet. He lost his fear of shadows, occasionally mentioning seeing them on the wall but no longer seeming afraid of them. He still exhibited a fear of the dark, though it did not stop him from going into the basement by himself. After a couple of months, none of the fears could be seen at all. He had watched a scary movie the previous week and was fine afterwards. He no longer went around locking everything at night.

He used to be clingy and fearful, but after the remedy he became happier, more content, more venturesome, and more confident. He can wait a longer period of time before looking for his mother. He hides less and is more confident out of doors. He doesn't panic any more.

His mother reports, "He is now more helpful and speaks more. He is eating a greater variety and has come out of his shell. He used to have no fear of injury whatsoever. He was indestructible, had no self-preservation instinct. As if he had no fears. He showed a kind of painlessness when he was injured, but after the remedy he began to react more to pain. Now if he falls he will cry. He has become a little cautious. He's careful going downstairs. It's as if he can now learn from his experiences."

## A Note to Doctors and Parents

I would like to plead, for the sake of the child, that the parents remove or limit potentially frightening situations from the child's life. While we

# STRAMONIUM

all **may** feel that we do this, it might be worthwhile for us to visualize the situation from a child's point of view, and not just any child, but in particular a *Stramonium* child. Whether your goal is to help your *Stramonium* child to heal, or whether it is to prevent your child from ever becoming a *Stramonium*— the same caution applies. **Limit exposure to television, videos, computer games, and stories that involve evil, that involve torture, that involve evil versus purity.** Many young children can handle nothing more than a simple version of good versus bad. This type of child has an antenna that will pick up ideas about evil and use the images to undermine himself. Even though you can not stop all such situations, you can limit them.

Let me end with a story that illustrates this point. One of my patients, a sweet little three year old girl, when I asked her what scared her most, told me her very biggest fear was of Mr. McGregor in the Peter Rabbit story. I mention this to show that when an antenna is out it will receive the exact signal it is searching for. And no matter how innocuous the thing that is feared may seem to be to an adult, it is a valid fear to the child. We all know that there is no way for us to completely protect a child from all frights, but we can make every effort to limit the exposure and thus offer some measure of protection.

# The Element of Violence

> Do not go gentle into that good night,
> Old age should burn and rave at close of day;
> Rage, rage against the dying of the light.
> Dylan Thomas, *Do Not Go Gentle into That Good Night*

Violence has long been associated with *Stramonium* and will be seen in many of the patients needing it. In some it will be the primary effect, while in others it may simply accompany their other complaints. If we look at it from a few different angles, we may discover why *Stramonium* children tend to gravitate toward this characteristic. We tend to think of *Stramonium* children as having violent behaviors. But violence does not limit itself to the emotional realm; it can be seen in any aspect of the child. *Emotional violence is only an example* of the many kinds of violence that belong to the segment of the *Stramonium* cycle called violent overreaction.

There are two things to keep in mind as you read this chapter: First, *Stramonium* has a strong tendency to exhibit a quick neurologic response to stimuli in the form of some violent overreaction. Second, violence may not be what the child intended or desired. It may simply be his way of responding to stress or to fear.

The case of Noah, a ten year old boy, illustrates how violence can sometimes be a response to stressful situations. Perhaps the place to begin is with Noah's parents. Bob, an irritable sort of person, is something of a workaholic. Although he himself does not drink, his father and three generations before him died of alcohol related illnesses. Alice is not only a doctor but also writes articles for magazines as well as doing some book editing. Their relationship was troubled, often on the brink of divorce. Then Alice got pregnant, and two months later she informed Bob, who promptly asked for a divorce. Alice says she was deeply shocked by this response.

While there are usually two sides to a story, the only side I heard was Alice's. She says that they separated right away, and their divorce became final when Noah was only six months old. Bob never set eyes on his son. Alice reports a difficult pregnancy, with vomiting throughout the whole nine months. In addition, she developed two kidney infections, one in the third month and another in the fifth. Her labor started a few weeks early, and after she spent a full day laboring and pushing, the midwife said the baby's head was too large and called for an emergency Cesarean section.

From the moment he came out Noah started screaming, and he never stopped. It turned out that his temperature and heart rate were too high, and suspecting meningitis, Alice's colleague performed a spinal tap, which came out negative. Eventually, the fever dropped and Alice was able to take Noah home. But she hated her baby. "I never bonded with him. How can you love someone who takes away love?" It was because of this baby that she had been robbed of her husband. She developed feelings of abandonment, loneliness, hatred, and guilt—all intermixed.

Noah's first year was uneventful except for a few coughs and colds, but after every vaccination during his first eighteen months, he would spike a fever and shriek for almost a week. Each time, the pediatrician feared meningitis and each time did a spinal tap, but after three taps came back normal, he stopped performing them.

Alice began to notice Noah's behavior taking a turn for the worse at about eighteen months. "He started to cry out in his sleep, screaming really. When I went near him, he would kick me. Then his eyes would open, but he looked terrified, as if he didn't recognize me. To this day Noah still has night terrors, only they have become more exaggerated with time.

"At about the same time that the night terrors began I noticed that he started to cling to me a lot. Whenever I left the room he would follow, and when we went out he would stay very close to me. He became so scared—scared of the whole world, it seemed. We couldn't watch television because he was terrified by something on every show, even the puppets on Mr. Rogers! I had to walk out of many a children's movie, carrying this screaming child. I began to feel more and more isolated because we couldn't go anywhere—invariably I would have to pick him up and run. At the zoo, the animals terrified him. At the fair, the children's painted faces made him scream and bury his face in my lap.

# THE ELEMENT OF VIOLENCE

"Worst of all were—and still are—the nights. He is so scared of the dark that he procrastinates over bedtime until finally I lie down with him. After a while he falls asleep, and then I can get up and go to my own bed, but in an hour or so the night terrors begin and they last for about a half hour. Sometimes he has several a night.

"When the dreams first began, Noah started to isolate himself. By two, at the age when other kids were checking each other out, he was either in my lap, or sitting alone in a corner of the room with a toy, or standing and staring out into space. He looked kind of dumb, which he is not—his tests showed him to have above average intelligence. And yet, the older he gets the more isolated he gets. Other children don't play with him. They ignore him. It's gotten to the point that he doesn't want to go to play group any more. In fact, he doesn't want to leave the house at all. I could rattle off a dozen fears he might come up with at any given moment. Mostly, he stays in his room or near me. Sometimes I actually find him under the bed or in the closet hiding—from what, I don't have the faintest idea.

"Now, along with everything else, he's developed a streak of violence. But the violence is only aimed at me. He screams, shrieks, kicks and bites, all the while yelling, 'Go away! I hate you! I'm gonna kill you! I'll set you on fire, I want to cut your throat!' And at this point he'll start to chase me and hit me over and over again. I often have to duck his abuse. This can go on for maybe thirty minutes, but then he begins to whimper and gets really apologetic and begs for hugs and his bottle. He tells me he loves me and makes me promise not to leave him. But in less than two hours he again starts screaming, 'Get away from me!' and he jumps up and slams the door to his room four or five times. Once he even broke it. He says that during these episodes 'A man takes me over and his name is Daddy.'

"You know why he chases me and threatens to kill me? Simply because I didn't do something just exactly as he expected. If what I do is not to his liking, he throws a temper tantrum and the whole thing begins again."

*Stramonium* 1M ended this cycle of violence and fear, and left the child in a grieving, sensitive mood. At this point counseling had its most dramatic effect, both on him and his mother.

# STRAMONIUM

## Violence as a reaction to being offended easily

As can be seen in Noah's story, at least one facet of *Stramonium* violence may be caused by sensitivity and sadness. His feelings can be hurt easily, and at any given moment he will strike out, sometimes because of poor impulse control, and sometimes because he cannot find the right words to express what he is feeling. "One thing that invariably triggers a violent outburst is someone saying something that hurts his feelings. He'll hit and yell and scream. He's unbelievably sensitive to the least little slight." To me, the symptom of offense leading to violence is expressed in the rubric: **MIND: Excitement, alternating with convulsions.**

## Violence as a reaction to having their world intruded upon

If the violence becomes all encompassing, it will increasingly color the child's whole experience. At that point, instead of just having occasional violent outbursts, he becomes irritable in many ordinary situations, especially when his space is somehow violated. For instance, one little girl was extremely crabby in the morning and would yell at her parents, "Get out of my room or I'll break your bones!" Strong words for a six year old girl. She used violence as a way to control others. Another child combined this with rudeness and withholding affection from his father. He would strike his father in the face whenever he tried to pick him up and hug him.

While some children react to the least offense, others take it one step further, by interpreting it as a deliberate personal insult. They are convinced the other person is doing this on purpose to hurt them. For example, one seven year old boy had a minor motor incoordination that made it a bit difficult for him to write or to play certain games. He became overly sensitive about his limitation and reacted aggressively to any imagined offense or opposition. His mother told me, "He will fist fight with friends if anything they say or do strikes his sensitive spot. That really hurts his feelings. He might take it out right away on the one who offended him, or he might hold it in and then later jump on his little sister and start hitting her. He dominates her every chance he gets, threatening and testing his strength against her. We have to pull him off of her." This child was using anger and temper tantrums as a way of controlling the whole family.

# THE ELEMENT OF VIOLENCE

If the child is younger, say two to four, he may bite other children whenever he does not get his way. Two year old Josh, who has respiratory infections and asthma, as well as many fears, can be quite domineering and obstinate. He tries in every way he knows to get what he wants, never giving up. But at a certain point, (a point at which other children this age would either control themselves or let out a few screams), Josh starts biting. He bites anyone who frustrates him, even the babysitter or the children at school.

When seven year old George gets a little too excited, he acts out by not listening, by moving around too much, by dancing, turning, and jumping. At that point he seems to lose awareness of his surroundings and to feel unsure of what others' expectations are of him or what he will get from them. For example, if his parents or teacher reprimand him with so much as a mild, "Stop that," he will erupt with frustration, anger, even rage, and start clawing, kicking, hitting, and threatening. He screams at his father, "If I could, I would break your bones!"

Add to this picture not just cruelty but also a bit of arrogance. The child begins to feel a bit above others. While this will not be a big part of the case, recognizing it can explain why some of these children seem so hard. The contempt they exude for those they hate, those who contradict them, those who intrude upon their world—is so strong and comes on so suddenly that they strike out without thinking.

One way to view this intolerance to intrusion or contradiction is as pure reaction. Picture for a moment a spring that has been compressed to the limit, then along comes some small object that knocks against it, and Snap! If you can look at the child's emotions in the same way, it will make it easier to see why the least contradiction or being touched or spoken to or picked up—any one of these 'insults'—can be like a missile hurled against this tightly coiled child. Snap! It triggers a volley of rage and fury, of kicking and punching. Clearly, there is no stopping him at that point. He is on automatic and therefore cannot respond to reason. For him, considering consequences is out of the question. This kind of rage can also erupt when there is an intrusion upon his sleep, such as any noise or touch. Even morning and daylight intruding on his sleep can be processed as an insult and reacted to with anger.

## STRAMONIUM

In the systems cycle for *Stramonium*, I perceive rage, fury, violence, and shrieking as belonging to one segment, one element in the loop. For this I have found the following rubrics useful: **MIND: Rage during convulsion; MIND: Irritability if spoken to; MIND: Irritability in the morning**; and **MIND: Touch, aversion to**. I think these all fit the picture of the tightly wound spring, so easily snapped and released, devoid of any control over impulses. *Stramonium* should be added (in italics at least) to the rubric: **MIND: Impulsive**.

### Violence as a reaction to fear

As mentioned in the *Fear* section and in the description of the cycle, there are situations in which the child who feels threatened or fearful will strike out. In these instances there is no real desire for violence or joy derived from it. It is an instinctive response. His feeling of being threatened overshoots into violence of some kind.

This may even be found in toddlers who lash out and scream and pull away—all due to fear. As they grow older, they may begin to bite or scratch when approached, but it is only because of fear. It is an automatic behavior that takes over as their mechanism to handle the fear that overwhelms them. After delivering the strikes, the child may seem as much the victim as his parent or sibling. If old enough and aware enough, he may feel confused, because he has no idea why others are shocked at his actions. Perhaps he feels that anyone facing a threat would have done exactly what he did. It is this type of *Stramonium* child who will grow increasingly withdrawn and introverted. Not knowing himself or the world, he feels uncomfortable with people and eventually can go into severe depression, which is the next segment of the cycle.

Sometimes the violence will come as a reaction to an immediate fear but it can also arise out of a past fright. Five year old Tyler was irritable, so irritable that he would constantly throw things or hit and kick others. This behavior began with a fright suffered some time ago, when he was accidentally locked in a bathroom by himself. At that same time he developed asthma, began to regress, and became overly meticulous about everything. These are all symptoms belonging to the *Stramonium* picture.

# THE ELEMENT OF VIOLENCE

## Violence as an unconscious reaction

Sometimes violence will be present but without the child being at all aware that he is being violent. In such situations the violence will not be directed toward any one person or object, but rather come as a random discharge, an explosion of destructive energy. That kind of reaction is the essence of this segment. At the end of this explosion, the child appears frayed and beaten, as do those observing it.

Another example of violence without meanness can be observed in some autistic *Stramonium* children. I once thought that violence would be a major characteristic in such children, but in fact, it tends not to be. Although I have certainly seen *Stramonium* autistic children who exhibited a fair amount of violence, more often it will not be the predominant feature. Rather, it is the detached, faraway, autistic qualities of the child—the shut off/dead segment—that will mostly point to *Stramonium*.

Mostly, violence will be seen in these children only when one tries to restrain them, or if they for some reason become frightened. But this will be a striking out for protection, rather than an expression of true violence. The effect, however, may be the same on the poor unwary intruder into their world, who finds himself suddenly attacked and bitten or clawed at fiercely.

In the *Sleep* section, there is a full description of violence without meanness as seen during night terrors. While the child is experiencing the night terror, he seems to be stuck between the unconscious world and the conscious world. While in that in-between state, he has no awareness of his present situation and so cannot correctly perceive his room or his parents or anything in his physical environment. His behavior indicates that he is probably experiencing fright, for he strikes out, tearing apart the bed, or hitting, scratching, and kicking his parents. All the while they are doing whatever they can to try to calm him down, but in his confusion, he seems to see it as an attack. This type of confusion is one of the key features of *Stramonium*. It is a fundamental segment, another element which fits into the dynamic cycle of this remedy's disorder. It is the nature of these segments to flow from one into the other. Thus, the night terror leads into the confusion, and the confusion brings on the fear that causes him to strike out.

In a sense, I view the type of violence which erupts from the unconscious in the same way as any of the neurologic explosions that *Stramonium* is so well known for. Therefore it does not surprise me when it comes up later in the interview that the child has seizures or other neurologic disorders. They are but another expression of the same aspect of the violence in the remedy. During a seizure, some children will actually begin to destroy furniture and scratch or strike out at anyone who comes near them. Similarly, a child in the throes of meningitis may not realize what he is doing and begin to bite or scratch those around him. The Tourette's syndrome child who needs *Stramonium* will also strike out uncontrollably, sometimes to his own consternation as well as that of his parents.

Another type of violence the child is not consciously aware of may be seen in the delirium accompanying high fevers or during an upper respiratory tract infection. Probably a part of the brain is affected by the infection, leaving him incapable of recognizing anything, or fearing for his life. The child becomes wild, rolling all over the bed, his head thrashing on the pillow, or he may scream and yell and run about, trying to find a way out of the labyrinth. The same behavior sometimes appears during a bacterial or viral meningitis, in which some children, due to fear, will run to their parents for protection or comfort. But it is also possible that a child will recognize no one, including his parents, and if they come into the room to try to calm him down, he will turn violent, raging and striking out because he feels he must escape from them. At such times, a small child can actually do a lot of damage, breaking or throwing things as he flails about in panic. This example illustrates the dynamics of the segment of overreaction (inflammation and fever) leading to confusion of self and reality, leading to fear, leading back to the segment of violent overreaction.

Let me stress that, while a number of *Stramonium* children may exhibit only the unconscious type of violence, in some the violent overreaction eventually seeps through to other facets of the child, not only producing twitches and jerks and other violent physical symptoms, but even transforming the personality. It is at this stage that you will see a conscious enjoyment of violence.

THE ELEMENT OF VIOLENCE

# REACTIVITY

### Sensory Integration/Motor Overflow

Between the conscious violence and the violence that is unconscious lies a violence that is the result of a motor overflow and the confusion that follows. Here we find the child not only having unconscious explosions but also becoming confused from too much sensory input, which causes him to react without thinking, sometimes violently. Different examples of motor overflow, such as falling out of a chair, are discussed in a separate section on concentration, but the focus here is on the frustration that comes out of confusion, causing the child to shift into a violent reaction.

Another way to say it is that the sensory/motor overflow makes the child confused, and that confusion contributes to his misinterpreting other people's motives. The irrational behavior that follows is especially difficult for other children to deal with. Children under five can often handle unpredictability in other kids, but older children will peg such a child as the hitter or the fighter or the troublemaker. They do not realize that he is not doing it on purpose, but rather out of a confusion that leads him to see a threat where none was made, or an offense where none was meant.

One day seven year old David became very agitated and scared at school, and began racing from one group to the next. No one knew exactly what had set off the agitation, but at one point as the class was moving to another room, he pushed the child ahead of him so he could be first in line. It was not long before things escalated. The child turned, to keep himself from falling, but David, thinking he had turned to hit him, pushed the child even harder. The teacher, trying to get to the bottom of it, asked him why he had done that. But David would not say anything, he just grinned and tried to hide. When the teacher tried to explain that he must wait his turn like everyone else, he hauled off and hit her. She picked him up to remove him for a time out, and he began to scream and kick and hit her wildly. At that point, they took him home. David simply did not understand. It took two hours and a lot of discussion for him to begin to formulate what had happened. It all started as a case of sensory overflow, too many inputs. In his excitement, he did not even realize he had pushed the child, so when the child turned, he thought he was going to hit him. David had acted intuitively to protect himself.

# STRAMONIUM

"David can't cope with free play time at all. For him, too many different things are going on. Another day, several children ran outside, and when he saw them, he ran screaming, 'I want to go out!' The teacher explained that those children had to come back in because it was not yet time for recess, but he kept on screaming, 'I want to go out! I want to go out!' all the while hitting and kicking. He did not calm down until they finally let him step out for a minute and then come back in." He had gotten stuck in that single idea and was unable to listen or to integrate anything else until he could act out the stuck thought.

This type of child seems to cave in under the slightest amount of stress. "Whenever he drops something or is unable to do some manual task, such as tying his shoelaces or manipulating a toy on his desk, he screams and cries. He has no frustration tolerance at all. That's why we send him late every morning to kindergarten, so he can miss the free play time, which is when these things most often happen."

This perseverative behavior that the child employs in an attempt to limit his confusion can lead to violence, for when the persistent action is interrupted or the ritual broken, the child becomes even more confused. Overwhelmed by confusion, he may resort to a temper tantrum and finally violence. For example, one mother said of her six year old, "Philip was four when these behaviors gradually began. One day at playtime, I picked out a toy and gave it to him, but he tossed it down and threw a temper tantrum. He was always having temper tantrums, many every day. That particular time it took a full twenty minutes before I understood that I had not given him the exact toy he had wanted. And when I tried to so much as touch him during that tantrum, he actually scratched me and even tried to bite me."

Sometimes the perseverative behaviors will take the shape of obsessive ideas about violence and weapons. For example, a child who obsesses over guns and swords and the bad people who use them is likely to turn anything, even a banana, into a gun, and then chase his siblings with it.

On the other hand, when sensory integration issues are at the root of the problem, the child may develop an identity crisis in which violence plays a role. This could happen, for example, in a child who is slightly confused about his surroundings and no longer is able to see a difference between himself and others. He will mimic the actions of whoever is nearby, and if that person happens to be aggressive, he too may become aggressive. He readily adopts whatever behaviors he sees. This also can occur in autistic children.

**Temper Tantrums**

Just as likely, a child will resort to temper tantrums when he feels overwhelmed, and may exhibit violence as part of the tantrum. Totally unable to sort out his feelings, he may fall to the ground, kicking and screaming. Should the parent attempt to enter into this spider web of heightened neural activity (a good way to picture the overreactive segment), the child instinctively becomes violent, kicking, scratching, and forcefully pushing away whoever approaches him. At times he will pick up whatever objects are in sight and throw them around.

As the child grows older, the temper tantrums may accelerate into rages. One mother said, "He tries to hurt me on purpose. He hits, bites, scratches, spits, throws things at me, or tears up his room over the least little thing. He especially likes to punch me in the face. But I can't tell if he really likes being that way. He seems to just act that way. Without thinking, he just starts hitting. But after the attack is over, he cries and wants me to hold him and not leave him. He begs pitifully to sleep in my bed." Three months after *Stramonium* 1M was given, the confusion and violence stopped, and he began to "come out of his shell and make friends."

So in one respect, the temper tantrums are a form of the mind getting stuck and not being able to process events. The child wants something and is so bent on getting it that, if denied, he is incapable of processing that bit of information (the denial). So, as a way of discharging his frustration, he resorts to a temper tantrum, either to delay, or to reject what was told him. If you have ever observed this kind of behavior, you can see how it fits the rubric: **MIND: Obstinacy.** While there are several other ways to use this rubric, it applies in situations such as this.

Five year old Sara suddenly started having temper tantrums, turning red in the face and screaming for what she wanted, crying hysterically and stomping on the floor. But when given what she hollered for, she would scream all over again, "No! No!" Apparently it was something else she wanted. During these episodes Sara would hit herself on her head or thighs, or bash anyone who came near her. She also at the same time developed night terrors. Every night she shrieked, wanting comfort, while in the daytime she developed new fears, of dogs and loud noises. When confronted with them she would start screaming. If someone yelled at her she would fall apart and become hysterical. Sara is a good example of a child who cannot process all the stimuli from her environment and so develops tantrums as a method of dealing with unexpected situations.

# THE JOY OF TERROR

There may be an addictive quality to violence. A small number of children seem to ultimately take great joy in hurting others or being violent. Of course, this occurs under various circumstances and may be justified by different rationales, but whatever the reason, the behavior is the same.

**The Policeman**

There is one type of child that I call 'the policeman'. He likes violence and will hurt his siblings whenever his parents seem angry at them. While this behavior is more common in other remedies such as *Hyoscyamus* and *Tuberculinum*, it is found in this remedy as well. If you happen to notice that the child hits reactively as soon as the parent lets him know there is a problem, it may help you to decide whether the child needs *Stramonium*. Eighteen month old Tyrone displays this kind of punishing behavior. He hits or bites his four and five year old siblings whenever their mother yells at them. I found it hard to believe that the little guy actually could do as much damage as the parents claimed, but when his siblings came into the consulting room and disrobed, I was shocked to find bite marks of that little mouth all up and down their backs. "He's the policeman of the family. If his brother does something that upsets us, sometimes Tyrone will grab his nipples and twist. It's the same with animals. He really likes them, but if an animal does anything wrong, he'll pull its ears." In this type of child, morality is intricately tied to consequence, and he will diligently mete out what he considers to be justice.

Even in a peaceful household in which the parents conscientiously limit exposure to the horrors of life, you may still see *Stramonium* aggressions. "One day," a father reports, "I walk into the kids' bedroom and find Clinton chasing his little sister. Anna is screaming, and he's growling and chasing her with a stick, really trying to hurt her. This wasn't the usual kid stuff. I asked what was going on and told him to stop it. He said he was Mr. McGregor and she was Peter Rabbit and he was going to stuff her into a pot." The boy had latched on to someone aggressive and emulated their aggressive behavior by becoming the villain in the Beatrix Potter story. Numerous reports from other parents reveal similar stories. So, even if you limit exposure, which parents should do, a child might still feel a thrill over something aggressive and begin to mimic it to vent his inner fears, and then rationalize it as the correct and fair thing to do.

I think one reason the child may exhibit sudden violence has to do with a need to feel important. It takes only a slight bit of arrogance to condone being brutally just and cruelly vindictive. Should haughtiness show up as a major part of the case, it will make it all the more difficult to differentiate between *Stramonium*, *Veratrum album*, *Tarentula hispanica*, *Hyoscyamus*, and *Platina*.

## Hyperactivity with gloating laughter

The *Stramonium* child who is hyperactive may show a combination of some of the attributes already mentioned: poor control of his impulses, overreacting, lack of awareness of what he is doing, and loving to be violent.

Perhaps the story of Bryan, a three year old, will help to illustrate this. Although a child's mother may offer a lot of information during the interview, the most helpful clues usually come from simply observing the child. When Bryan's mother and I first start talking, he is sitting there on her lap, playing with a gray toy dog. At this point it could be any remedy. But after just a minute he too begins to talk, and his voice grows louder and louder, drowning out the adult conversation. He is obviously not talking to anyone in particular, just looking at the wall, and in an unfocused flow, yelling over our escalating voices. He then focuses on one subject after another and begins to discourse, as if the adult conversation does not count, or more significantly, as if there is no such conversation.

Now some restlessness sets in and he begins to rock back and forth on a ball, babbling loudly to himself, totally ignoring any questions put to him. After a while, he starts rocking a little faster, and puckering his lips with effort, seems engaged in some project with his stuffed toy dog. Finally he succeeds in yanking off its front paw. The mother interjects, "He loves to do horrible things like that!" After this destructive act, he starts laughing a fiendish laugh, a long "Uhhh, huh huh huh. Uhhhhh, huh huh huh huh huh," again and again as his mother tries to put the paw back on the puppy. As he laughs one can see by his twisted grin and the cunning look in his eyes that he knew perfectly well what he was doing when he delimbed the defenseless dog.

Soon he starts biting the dog, all the while laughing that laugh and making depraved sounds of enjoyment. He moans, "Uhhhhh," and then bites the dog and then goes back to his moaning "Uhhhhh," once again. After repeating this several times, he again begins to rock back & forth, then abruptly turns his attention to the toy dog, this time trying to decapitate it as well as ripping off its limbs.

By now I am thinking I have seen the full extent of torture he could possibly inflict on the pup (and am feeling relieved that it is only a stuffed animal), but in a final grand gesture he holds it up by its one remaining paw, and with a wicked grin on his face, starts twirling it around and around in a dizzying, torturing way. It takes but a small step of the imagination to visualize a few scenes from the parents' stories about what he does to live animals, siblings, parents, friends, and strangers.

Watching this behavior and the cunning look on his face, it occurs to me that he is consciously trying to disrupt the office visit, though it is not quite as obvious as it would be in *Tuberculinum, Veratrum album, Tarentula hispanica* or *Lachesis*.

By now the distressed mother has replaced the dog's limbs, but, undaunted, Bryan rips them right off again with that diabolic laugh and starts rocking again. He rocks throughout the interview, sometimes so hard that his mother has to pin him to the chair. He clearly wants to escape, and it is only her grip that keeps him from bolting. He struggles and protests and then gives in, protests again and gives in again, and finally throws a tantrum.

The mother tries as calmly as possible to continue the interview. "We have quite a few behavior problems with this boy. He is restless. He doesn't like to sit and eat, he'd rather rush around. He seems to have a lot of energy, always climbing and swinging on things. He is very mischievous. I think

## THE ELEMENT OF VIOLENCE

he likes to stir people up and do things he shouldn't. Sometimes he'll hug us, but soon after that he'll punch us or push and shove other kids and then start laughing.

"He doesn't have a best behavior. He's always destructive in stores. It is as if there is a monster on the outside with a little sweet boy underneath. No matter what we try, the monster is growing and the sweet boy is shrinking. The monster is taking over. We dread going out in company. He goes completely bonkers. We always end up chasing after him and restraining him. That's what our evenings out are like."

In the office he is both contrary and oppositional. Whenever his mom says "Be quiet, I can't concentrate," he gets louder. She says that whenever she tells him not to do something that involves hurting someone, he immediately will do it. When let loose in the office, he runs about, gleefully grabbing everything he can get hold of. He fidgets and fidgets, and when restrained, he eyes the plants, points at them, and babbles loudly. All this, interspersed with guttural laughter.

He never stops trying to get off the chair, and when his mother holds him down, he kicks and bites her, screaming as if possessed. As the interview continues, she has to hold him tighter and tighter and keep saying, "Calm down. Calm down."

Whenever the mother loosens her grip, he flies off to get at the computer, then runs back to rock on the chair, then shoots off again to tear the plant to bits, then back again to rock. The child is totally out of control.

As they are leaving, he shifts into full gear, touching everything, grabbing his genitals, throwing papers and books on the floor, moving faster and faster like a tornado, destroying everything in his path—all the while laughing that horrid laugh and dangling limp wrists like a praying mantis.

The destructiveness has greatly increased over time. He started out just tearing apart his stuffed animals and dolls, but now he breaks every toy he owns. In fact, anything that captures his attention is fair game and will eventually be destroyed. The cordless telephone has been replaced numerous times, as have the VCR and the television. All their plants have suffered amputations. And while the father is describing this, the boy, as if to confirm it, gleefully amputates the dog's paws once again, tossing them across the room and laughing his guttural laugh. While this is a rather extreme case of *Stramonium* hyperactivity, it is worth studying because it contains all the ingredients I wanted to point out. Bryan's story illustrates how restlessness, violence, acting out and destructiveness are all different examples of the same fundamental segment. To a certain extent they are interchangeable.

Many children have these hyperactive tendencies, sometimes accompanied by a violence that is explosive and reactive. Six year old Juan is one such child. His mother complains that he is wild. If she tries to set limits or restrain him in any way, he punches her in the genitals. When he goes into rages, he looks and acts as if possessed. When the wild look comes over his face, his pupils dilate, and his face and ears turn red. He becomes very aggressive, kicking and striking his parents, spitting on them, or choking various family members. The parents are actually frightened by these attacks. When he is at his best, he is unruly and uncontrolled.

Sometimes this violence is perpetrated just for the joy of it, sort of as a by-product of the hyperactivity, as in *Hyoscyamus*. In such cases the mother will say, "He is a showoff in front of other children and always pushes younger kids around just for the attention it gets him. He enjoys it."

## The end result

As the child is drawn further and further into the world of violence, he is less and less able to comprehend the rules and morals that constitute normal behavior. He grows to relish violence in any form. He is drawn to it in books, in films, and on television. He becomes violent just for the fun of violence, enjoying torturing those around him. This enjoyment of his has an edge of arrogance, but not as great as that of *Tarentula hispanica* or *Hyoscyamus*. Because of this contempt for others he feels free to disobey anyone, especially his mother, and is abusive to others with no fear of punishment. A good point of differentiation is that the *Hyoscyamus* child may focus his violence on the next youngest sibling, whereas *Stramonium* can be violent to anyone. But this is not the usual *Stramonium* state; it is rather uncommon to see such a deeply pathologic level. When the child is still in the early phases he will only be violent as a protective mechanism, later only as an impulse, but eventually he will be violent on purpose. It is the easy option. In fact, he may actually feed on violence, dreaming of it, writing about it, drawing horrid pictures, and acting it out.

# THE ELEMENT OF VIOLENCE

## Observing the Joy of Violence

The enjoyment of violence may be seen in a child's expression or in how he talks about violence or reacts to it. In a conversation with eight year old Max I asked, "What do you do if someone hurts your feelings?" He replied, "I jump on their bones...I love to fight...I like fist fights." His pleasure was evident in the look on his face when he watched violent shows or played violent games, making anything into a lethal weapon, even a piece of bread or his shoes.

When his mother was asked what about Max bothered her the most, she replied, "He embarrasses me in public. He won't listen, and does really mean things to other children." One example of the meanness was his deliberate attempt to dump a baby out of its cradle. And in my office, he hurled the books on my desk against the wall and jabbed his mother's arm with a pen. These were but a few of his outrageous behaviors.

You can often assess whether a child is in this phase by observing the fiendish grin on his face or the evil sounding laugh that erupts as he struggles to escape the stronghold of his parent. He obviously enjoys his own behavior. Violence will also be apparent in the pictures these children draw or the way they destroy their toys or turn them into weapons. Even the clothes they wear may display images of darkness and evil, or violent words.

## Self-Directed Violence

*Stramonium* children can also turn the violence on themselves, as they head toward the next segment, the element of closing off. Sometimes the force of sheer emotion will break through as impulsive actions against others, but it just as soon can find an outlet in self-destructive tendencies. Children as young as one month or as old as eight years may throw intense temper tantrums if they do not get their own way, or when they are hungry or tired. This can be from a purely oppositional behavior. In this mood, a child may turn on himself, banging his head on the floor or scratching his face, gouging his skin, or hitting his head with his fists. He may even stab his pants and thighs with a pen or pencil, as does *Lyssinum*. And yet, if admonished, he will weep like the little child he really is.

Just as children sometimes impulsively hit bystanders out of frustration, so too they may turn the violence on themselves when frustrated, angry, or if contradicted. Four year old Allison gets into rages when things do not go her way, kicking and punching others but also smacking herself on the head very hard. She can be quite mean to other kids and yet is sweet as can be with cats.

As these children grow into teens, the violence may become more controlled, more suppressed. They still feel the anger inside but they hold it in. What seems to be operating at this point is a fear of confrontation combined with a feeling that it is their fault, that there is something wrong with them, and this makes them feel isolated.

At times they will become upset with themselves because they are unable to achieve what they visualized. This may evoke a temper tantrum during which they end up destroying the thing they were working on. And it might not stop there. Some will kick the floor so hard it must hurt, or rip their clothes, or more rarely, tear out clumps of their hair.

This violence enacted on themselves often arises from an overexcited nervous system. At first, the only clue may be the way the child claws at himself when scratching his eczema. Later on, he may start biting his nails. At another time he may inflict injury upon himself in the middle of a temper tantrum. As it progresses, he will begin to hit his head on purpose. Finally, he may cut himself with razors or say that he wishes he were dead.

**After the Remedy**

After the remedy, the need for violence diminishes and becomes a non-issue. This may be observed in different ways, from better impulse control, to understanding the possible repercussions of his actions, to less show of violence in the games he plays.

This was true in four year old Ryan, who was hyperactive, malicious, and fond of hurting others, most especially his father, whom he hated. After the remedy he was happier and interacted better with siblings and classmates, but especially with his father. Immediately upon entering the office they thanked me profusely. "Since the remedy, he's a new boy. He's much more loving to his father. He even asks him for kisses. There's truly a remarkable change in his temperament. He's nice and calm and a lot more fun to be around. He comes up and hugs his father and says 'I love you.' He actually runs from his bed to hug his father goodbye as he's leaving for work. He's so pleasant to be around now, and he's the most obedient he's ever been. He'll do almost anything you ask him to."

However, this change did not happen overnight. Several months after the remedy, he still could not sit through a meal. Then, a few more months passed before his hyperactivity cut back considerably. That was years ago, and today his attitude toward his parents, especially his father, continues to be great.

After the remedy, parents often say their child has become sweeter, gentler, more affectionate. "Only once after the remedy did he do his make-believe violence, taking coat hangers and pretending they were guns. What a vast improvement! It was as if that sweet child had been switched off but is once more switched on. He even wants to read and draw again. And such a change in his pictures! They used to be of monsters, ghosts, devils, and werewolves, but now he draws the family or nature pictures.

"After the remedy the violence stopped. He is more gentle, more cautious, not suicidal like he was. He's out of his shell and is playing with other children better, not being mean to anyone or biting or hitting any longer. He is less feisty and angry, more low key."

I think it is important here to include a case management note for the homeopath. Some children you see will seem to fall somewhere in between two remedies and you will need to make a decision between the two. One such common dilemma is the choice between *Stramonium* and *Medorrhinum*. Though this was discussed briefly in the introduction and will receive fuller treatment in my book on hyperactivity, I would like to mention one point here. It is essential that you treat the more severe symptoms first. These will usually be the top layer. Since *Stramonium* possesses the more intense state of the two, if both states seem to be equally indicated, *Stramonium* should be given first. It has been my experience that if *Medorrhinum* is given first instead, you may see the child's overall health improve, but he becomes more violent. He may have fewer coughs and colds but now he screams a lot and has become aggressive, hitting other kids. This behavior is a sure sign that the remedies were given in the incorrect order.

If that should happen, *do not wait* for the next follow-up visit or for the *Medorrhinum* to stop acting. Prescribe *Stramonium* right away to diminish the violent outbursts. Later, at the appropriate time, give *Medorrhinum*.

## STRAMONIUM

The same thing holds true if you give any wrong remedy. Let us say that a *Stramonium* child is given *Lycopodium* or *Sulphur* or *Calcarea phosphorica* by mistake. While a few of his symptoms may improve, the child is likely to develop some violence or fears or other symptoms that are an exaggeration of the state he is in. This should be a clue that the case is suppressed. If this happens, the *Stramonium* symptoms will become more evident, more exaggerated. *Stramonium* should be given then, and the symptoms will disappear in short order.

# *The Element of Attention Difficulties*

**Introduction**

Hyperactivity and/or attention difficulties are a common presenting complaint these days for a growing number of children. This chapter will focus on some of the behaviors frequently noted in these children and discuss the different reasons behind the hyperactivity and inattentiveness. A more thorough description of the treatment of this disorder will be found in my forthcoming book on the topic, but for now let me just say that there is no one typical picture. Some of the children diagnosed with attention difficulties will be hyperactive, some will not. Some will show aggressiveness or violence or a lack of impulse control, but others will have none of these symptoms. In some you will see dullness or listlessness, but you might also see tics or seizures. All of these symptoms can occur in any combination, as seen in the children we will meet in this chapter.

**Restlessness/Hyperactivity**

The restlessness, or hyperactivity, that is so often found in *Stramonium* I believe to be a part of an overall nervous system excitability belonging to the violent overreaction segment. In its early stages, it finds an outlet in simple restlessness but later expresses itself through impulsive actions, violence, rage, or seizures. At first, however, only the restlessness will be evident. This compelling need to move is probably caused by an overly excited nervous system. That would explain why the child is so easily aggravated by any kind of excitement. Further, if the nervous system should become stretched beyond a certain point, the excitement will by-pass mere restlessness and produce soft neurologic signs, such as tics, grimaces, and involuntary motions of the hands. It seems that the more excitement the child feels, the more he will tic, and the more facial grimaces and hand gestures he will make.

# STRAMONIUM

It is easy to imagine why a constant state of fear can also lead to restlessness. This reaction may simply be a flight aspect of the 'fight or flight' syndrome. The child feels restless and flighty. After a while the restlessness may snowball, and then he will show signs of not being able to focus on what is happening around him and to him.

Restlessness may even be seen in an infant who does not stay asleep but tosses and turns all night long, or in a toddler who likes nothing better than to climb out of his crib or playpen or to romp all over the furniture. He never rests, and the tired mother has to constantly watch him to prevent accidents. She may also tell you that whenever it is necessary to hold him down, she can feel his muscles harden up and he may become rigid, as if waiting to spring free so he can race about again.

When the *Stramonium* child enters the school scene, he rarely is able to perform well, due to his excessive restlessness. He can sit at his desk and work quietly for short periods of time, but as the restlessness creeps over him, he quickly loses interest in whatever he's doing and keeps popping up. He may even try to continue the task while standing up or on the move. He fidgets and has to touch everything, just like *Veratrum album* and *Tarentula hispanica*. Because of his disruptive behavior, he may have to sit next to the teacher or be restrained in other ways. In the long run, he becomes the focus of frequent parent/teacher conferences.

One mother said, "He eats and drinks in a rush and then runs off to play. That's how he handles everything. He's always on the go. He races into his room then races out and bumps into his sister who starts to cry, but he just keeps on going as if he is not aware that there's any problem. He flies out of bed in the morning and goes full speed until night overtakes him."

For such a child, there's no rest, day or night. Even in bed he tosses and turns, grinds his teeth, and flips from one side to another. There's no stopping, no rest, no calm. He may even keep the action going by walking in his sleep. It's as if his nerves are firing off a message: Go! Go! Go!

As would be expected, exciting events make this kind of child's restlessness much worse. Whenever guests or new children come to the house he becomes unruly, loses all control, and runs around throwing things. Whenever the family is getting ready for a trip or some special occasion, he acts out more and more, bouncing off walls, making faces, joking, and shrieking. It's

# THE ELEMENT OF ATTENTION DIFFICULTIES

very clear that he thinks he is being quite funny.

One mother reported, "When we are about to leave a place that he likes, he gets very agitated and starts to misbehave. He runs around yelling, making faces, and twitching. If I catch hold of him, he immediately throws a temper tantrum. When he gets like this, it seems as if he stops being rational. He just wants what he wants when he wants it."

*Stramonium's* restlessness will sometimes be only purposeless—running and laughing and fooling around for no apparent reason. Or it may be purposeless *and* destructive. In such cases the child, as he runs about, may knock books off the bookcase, tear curtains, and pull paintings off the wall. But he is not doing it maliciously.

Sometimes the restlessness will actually be on purpose, and the child will deliberately run away from the parent, or dart off to fetch something he wants or to do something he is not allowed to do. The fact that he is crossing the street and his mother is yelling, "STOP," at the top of her lungs seems not to penetrate at all. He runs with abandon, in a world of his own. In fact if his mother tries to stop or even curb the restlessness, or to hinder the child in any way, he may become angry or violent, struggling at first just to break her hold on him. But after a bit he may kick and strike her or perhaps break down in a crying fit. I see the restlessness, anger, violence, and crying fits all as different expressions of the overreaction segment.

Four year old Ruthie offers an example of deliberately destructive hyperactivity. The entire time during the interview, her mother had to restrain her on her lap. The child at first squirmed a little but seemed happy. However, after several minutes she made it clear she 'wanted out' of the chair. But the mother held her fast. Undaunted, Ruthie began to tug and push, cry and scream, and finally she tried to hit her mother. When none of this worked, she threw a tantrum. At this point the mother said, "When she doesn't get her way, Ruthie acts like a wild animal." [And indeed she did spit at her mother.] "But if I let her do whatever she wanted, your whole office would be a disaster area."

When Ruthie finally got free, she proved her mother right. First she tore the papers on my desk, then threw my appointment card holder on the floor, then led her mother on a merry chase around the office. The whole time she was laughing a very strange laugh.

# STRAMONIUM

## Aggression

Violence is an easy habit to fall into for the *Stramonium* child. In some it will be episodic while in others it will show up with some sort of consistency. The hyperactive *Stramonium* child may act out aggressively for a number of reasons: poor impulse control, reactivity, being unaware of his actions, and/or simply loving to be violent.

In a child with poor impulse control, a perceived insult is responded to instantaneously, either by biting, kicking, and scratching, or by breaking things. Because so many events are interpreted by him as insults or injuries, such behaviors take place on a regular basis.

Sometimes a boy, not realizing that his sister is playing with a toy, will step up and take it. When his sibling shouts in protest, he may respond by striking out at her, completely unaware that it was he who was at fault in the first place. This kind of reactivity is also seen in these children when a playmate responds to their unconscious actions in a way that they interpret as hostile.

Violence often manifests in children who have poor attention. Part of the problem is that the child's lack of attentiveness prevents him from understanding his surroundings or from knowing what is expected of him. So when something takes him by surprise, he lashes out.

There are still other hyperactive children who show aggression for the sheer joy of it. While at first the violence is merely a by-product of the hyperactivity, the child begins to enjoy the attention it gets him, as does *Hyoscyamus*.

Violence may also erupt simply because a child does not get what she wants, as in the case of Ruthie. She was clearly bent on destruction, and when hindered, became violent. But there are other possible scenarios. For instance, a child may be so set on staying at the park that when that focus is interrupted, he becomes violent. Then often a tug of war will ensue, until finally the parent must lift the child and carry him, screaming and kicking, to the car.

With such children, this battle of wills goes on every day. The child hyperfocuses on one topic or one desire and will often first try to negotiate getting his way. Now, at this point there is a great temptation for the parents to give in. They know that the child will not act out and bounce all over the house as long as he is playing his video game or watching a movie he likes, so they often take the path of least resistance and give in. But there

## THE ELEMENT OF ATTENTION DIFFICULTIES

are times when the parent, for various reasons, cannot accommodate the child's wishes, and it is at those times that he will become violent.

Many children who are diagnosed with attention difficulties have a motor overflow problem which causes them to get tangled up in the stimuli they experience. A child who is very sensitive to noise will act out just from being in a noisy environment. As he becomes more and more restless, he will start to do things that are disruptive. Similarly, having too much company may make some children act hyper or silly.

### Unrelenting/Perseverative behavior

One aspect of focus disorders is that the child will be unable to keep his mind on one thing, but he can also shift gears and overfocus on one thing, and that may lead him into repetitive actions. The problem seems not to be that they cannot focus, but rather that they can't control it. In the same child there can be a shifting back and forth between lack of focusing and excessive focusing. This helps to explain why the same child will come home with a very good grade one day and a failing grade the next.

Inattentive behavior can, in time, lead to ritualistic or perseverative (repeatedly performing the same action over and over again) behavior. The inattentiveness signals an inability to focus, and the child at that stage may indulge in daydreaming, but that same child might become so focused at times that it turns into monomania. He cannot tolerate a single restriction or interruption. At that time, if the parents ask him to do something or not do something, or to come with them (in short, to cease what he is doing) he cannot obey. He will resist. He is compelled to resist. This inability to accept anything other than his present wish is a kind of rigidity, which often leads to a battle of wills between parent and child.

However, if the child has established a fair amount of impulse control, he may start out by trying to negotiate a deal with the parent. At first he may offer arguments, but as the tug of war escalates between the strength of his desire and the strength of the parent, he will resort to begging and pleading. If it then becomes apparent to him that he is not going to get what he wants, he becomes antsy and his loudness and restlessness increase.

For the longest time he may try to ignore his parents and disregard what they are telling him to do. This is the disobedience route, in which the child decides that his wishes are more important, and he blatantly carries them out without giving a hoot about what the parent wishes. It's as if he's saying to himself, "So what if Mom hollers at me? At least I'll get to play my game a little longer."

This relentlessness may also be apparent during the interview, as he talks louder and louder, not really directing it toward anyone in particular, just staring at the wall and yelling, until someone finally removes him from the scene.

It may be difficult for the child to focus on people or things because of this unrelenting quality. Lost in his thoughts, he may break something just because he is not aware of the surroundings or not paying attention to what he is doing. Conversely, he may hyperfocus on some object (unfortunately, it may be the telephone or the fax machine) and play with it doggedly until eventually it breaks.

Even the sexual acting out of these children may have an unrelenting quality. As in *Bufo*, *Hyoscyamus*, and in *Origanum*, the *Stramonium* hyperactive toddler's masturbation, when present, may be intense and of long duration. He may seem to be in a heated state as he rocks back and forth, back and forth.

**Poor impulse control**

In a child with attention difficulties you will often see *poor impulse control*. The child who is ruled by fears may start out by reacting with violence, and at this stage his impulses will be merely protective mechanisms. But as his disorder progresses, the impulse to strike may become the easiest option, or he may actually learn to enjoy violence and incorporate it into his daydreams, stories, and art work.

This child's life may be *quite chaotic*. His clothes are dirty, he loses his schoolwork, and his room is a mess. In a word, his outside world actually reflects the lack of order inside his mind. When asked to find something or to clean his room, he will tell you that he does not know how. He cannot focus properly due to all the chaos. Some children may also appear dull, and when dullness and a chaotic mental state mingle with restlessness, the child turns into one massive impulse, reacting to any and all stimuli with either confusion or violence or some silly act.

# THE ELEMENT OF ATTENTION DIFFICULTIES

The *lack of consistency* in his life may also be seen in his work. Sometimes he performs well, completes his task, and even does it with a perfectionistic flair. At other times he completely misses the point of the work and cannot keep up at all. Such a lack of consistency is bound to make the child hesitate before acting, sort of frozen in the same old dilemma of not knowing what to do. This capriciousness will plague him regarding not only big issues like how to spend the summer, but also in little things like what to wear for school or what game to play. This is a push-pull kind of existence.

Eventually the child may feel so defeated by life, so torn apart by vacillation, and so miserable from not catching on, that he will start saying he is no good and that he will never be 'right'. He may even begin to talk about killing himself. These episodic depressions seem to accompany the realization that he has failed once again.

## The Joker

More often than not the hyperactive *Stramonium* will be a joker. In keeping with the rest of the *Stramonium* picture, he may show a cruel kind of humor, playing practical jokes that he finds funny, but which are actually mean and hurtful to others. But there is another side to him, the happy practical joker, the clown, who makes a little joke and then laughs and laughs. It's easy for him to get into a happy mood, and in that mood he will act out and find it very funny, doubling over with laughter at his own actions. Once he is caught up in it, it may be hard to stop him. He does not understand that his actions are inappropriate, that he is causing trouble, and that he needs to contain himself a bit. You cannot help but be struck by the dramatic shift from a child who is so unhappy, violent and throwing tantrums to a happy, playful jokester. This excitement is rather immature in nature in that it tends to be funny to him and him alone. At such times he actually seems much younger than his age, and if seen at this time might be confused with a *Baryta carbonica* child.

A variation of this is the child who, caught up in his joy of the moment, will talk and talk, chattering to himself while playing or singing, as he runs around. Often he will talk loudly, drowning out his friends and parents. He might make up words or languages, even though he is six or seven years old. While loquacity is more commonly seen in other remedies such as

*Lachesis* and *Hyoscyamus*, it can be found in *Stramonium,* mostly during the manic phase.

I believe that this kind of excitability and exuberance fits into the violent overreaction segment of the *Stramonium* cycle alongside of other forms of stimulation such as violence and other manifestations of nervous system excitement. In this respect it shares some symptoms with *Hyoscyamus*. The difference is that for *Stramonium* it is simply excitability, whereas for *Hyoscyamus* it is an excitability of the limbic system of the hypothalamus, and therefore the joking is more likely to center upon sexuality and other strong drives. This trait of *Hyoscyamus* has a strength to it that is not easily confused with the *immature* joking of *Stramonium*.

## Dullness/Poor Concentration

Attention difficulties may be a primary complaint as far back as the birth of the child or ever since some shock occurred. The child may be inattentive at all times, or most of the time, or just episodically. Much of this description might be more appropriate to the **Autism** section, but I have chosen to place it here because so much of the literature currently available places all of these separate issues under one label—attention deficit disorder or attention deficit with hyperactivity. In reality the hyperactivity belongs to the violent overreaction segment, and the poor attention due to confusion belongs to the extreme shut down segment and also to the confusion segment.

A story we commonly hear in our practice is that the dullness of the child was first noticed following some surgery in which anesthesia was administered. Nine year old Eric's regression began in this way. Eric was only two and a half when he had surgery to correct a hernia. His mother told me, "He has not been the same since then. It became hard for him to grasp new concepts. For a while, he even lost his ability to speak properly. He was no longer on a par with the rest of his friends whereas, before, he had been quite bright. He even began to behave in a somewhat immature fashion. But we had him tested and he does have a normal IQ. It's just that whenever he gets frustrated, he starts to act childish and to overreact. At times he talks like a baby and makes up his own language, or he may speak in incomplete sentences and make mistakes in gender. They say he is dyslexic. Eric has taken to calling himself stupid because he is nine and can't read. Also, he has become very fearful of the dark."

# THE ELEMENT OF ATTENTION DIFFICULTIES

The reports from school may be quite bad. They say that he cannot learn, that he is unable to study, that he cannot retain anything, and that he refuses to do his schoolwork, wanting to play instead. He has a very short concentration span, maybe a few minutes. During the interview he does not pay any attention to questions put to him. His mother says the same thing happens at school.

"It's hard to make him sit down for long. He may try to do something and concentrate, but after a few minutes he is up and off." As the interview continues I can observe this same behavior. "Sometimes he fails because he gets so easily distracted at school, either by noise or by what the other boys are doing." Free time at school poses problems for many of these children. Eric is no exception. He becomes unruly when there are too many stimulating activities.

I noticed these things by observing him throughout the interview. At times I saw a faraway look as if he were not present. His parents say that he stares like that a lot and does not even snap out of it when they call him. After drifting away for a while, he may come back, but then will answer incoherently or incorrectly. Even in the middle of a sentence he may space out and get stuck in a thought or on a word, and the sentence will end right then and there.

When asked to do something, it is likely that he will forget. When asked a question, it is possible that he may not hear it. He appears to be in a trance or possibly contemplating something profound, but when asked what he is thinking about, he frequently will not answer.

Another parent of a five year old says, "As a toddler, Mikey learned everything very fast, drew quickly and accurately, and wrote his letters perfectly. He used to be a very good student and was advanced in math and English. But ever since the pneumonia he is slow. His writing skills have degenerated. He became dyslexic, transposing letters. He now speaks with difficulty, sometimes seeming slightly backward. He can't pronounce certain letters like L, M, or W. As he became more emotional he even began to stutter. He used to show promise in school and now he is behind. But happily, the remedy had a major effect on Mikey," and the father reports that his speech has improved. "It used to be all confused, a kind of tangled gibberish really. Only now, by comparison, can we see how bad it was."

## STRAMONIUM

As mentioned in the *Violence* chapter, motor overflow and confusion may be brought on by sensory integration difficulties, which can lead to problems in concentration, a shortened attention span, and slowness in comprehension. This can exist with or without hyperactive traits. The motor overflow leads to confusion which makes the child misunderstand the words or actions of others and take offense where none was meant. Such a child is also easily frustrated by the slightest amount of stress, especially when he realizes that he cannot write or draw something or use a kitchen utensil, or do something requiring fine motor skills.

A common strategy for limiting this confusion is to resort to perseverative behavior. The child becomes obstinate. He wants one thing and one thing only. If you should interrupt him, it may make him lose the one and only focus he had, thus driving him into further confusion. Another problem that can arise from putting all his attention onto one thing alone is that he misses out on all the other activities or events going on around him. He stays stuck in that one place.

### Conclusion

One last word on the dullness. I believe it may be a reaction to fear, a way of lulling himself into a state where the fears become subdued. An extreme picture of this can be found in the *Autism* section. Another possibility is that the dullness is a kind of confusion that comes on from feeling under the gun, which causes the brain to scramble and panic, not knowing what to attend to first.

There is another possible reaction to feeling threatened—hyperactivity, which is the flip side of dullness. When this happens, I believe that the nervous system has geared up to the point where restlessness takes over and forces him to act, often in an impulsive manner.

Even though attention difficulties are found in *Stramonium*, they are much more commonly seen in other remedies. Because of this sharing of symptoms, careful scrutiny is required in order to get the prescription right. The most essential step is to find the reason behind the symptoms, to discover the thing that brought about this state in the first place. *Only when we find out why certain symptoms exist can we determine which remedy will heal those ills.*

# *The Element of Closing Off; Introversion*

This is the water. Cold and black
It hurries in, it hurries back,
It never stops. And I wait long,
Perhaps to hear a gull's mad song
Or even wind. But not a noise
Breaks in upon this white hell's poise.
Only the water's lapping slack,
The silent blaring rush of black.

    Jeenet Lawton, from "To the Arms of The Sea"

Though not commonly thought of in relation to *Stramonium* children, I consider introversion to be a keynote, for much the same reasons put forward in the **Fear** and **Violence** sections. As the violence wreaks havoc within the child, as energy is wildly expended, there comes a time when the child must close off in order to clamp down on that energy, forming the closing off segment of the cycle. In the prolonged battle of the conscious versus the unconscious one possible outcome is that the child, being shell-shocked by the battle, becomes unsure of how to act, and so withdraws and goes inside. The children in this subset of *Stramonium* are either very introverted all the time, or simply have periods of introversion. Less intense than the violent *Stramonium*, these children may have been aggressive and outgoing in the past but have become introverted suddenly or over a period of time.

One type of introverted *Stramonium* is the child that has been abused or neglected. The abuse begins a process in which fear strikes at the heart of the psyche, leaving the child fearful, forsaken, and open to injury at any time. And so he turns inward and perhaps becomes hypervigilant. This kind of child has a poor self concept and cannot make friends. He lacks the social skills of knowing how to communicate with others and so is quiet and withdrawn. It is this type of introverted child that will most closely resemble an autistic child, or might even be mistaken for a *Natrum muriaticum* or *Staphysagria*. *Shy, reserved, unsure, and quiet, he seems to be in a world of his own.*

In another *Stramonium* type, the introverted sensitivity may be related to the child's own perceptions. Even though the parents may try to build up the child's self esteem, he does not respond. For all practical purposes, the child appears to be in a world of his own choosing. This mood grows, inhibiting his ability to express himself out in the world. Perhaps it is this isolation that leads older teens and adults to report an extreme sense of loneliness, of feeling forsaken by the world. "Like a lone soldier, hacking away at the enemy, absolutely alone, unable to talk to anyone. There is no one out there for me." It is easy to imagine these children and teens drifting more and more into their own world. After being so locked up within their minds, they begin to be dominated by delusions, which are always just around the corner for such children. "People scared me but I could always talk to the demons. I knew how to talk to them."

Not all these introverted children become delusional. But it is clear that the longer they remain introverted, and the more secluded they become, the more likely it is that delusions will arise, and their experience of that strange world will become magnified. Such a child starts out watching life as if it were a spectator sport, but because he is so deeply alone, he crosses over from watching to interacting, and begins to give in to impulses, but inappropriately. For example, he may be very shy with adults or strangers, yet be openly violent with members of his family, even to the point of punching them, sometimes as early as the age of three.

In time, as they keep vacillating between being extroverted and violent and being closed, sullen and incommunicative, they become less predictable. It is their strongly impressionable nature that causes them to close off, to isolate themselves. In either case, the child opens himself up to his unconscious, where he either feels terror or feels himself becoming the terror. I think of it as a child that is temporarily possessed, and yet is still able to experience what is happening to him. He senses the response others have toward him when he becomes the terror, but once he comes out of that state, he feels devastated, trying to understand what just occurred. He cannot understand it. He cannot fathom why people that he loves and trusts would feel so

## THE ELEMENT OF CLOSING OFF; INTROVERSION

badly toward him. And so now, in this subdued state, he once again becomes introverted. Why? Because he is so overwhelmed by a whirlpool of emotions: exhaustion (from his recent experience), bewilderment (from the struggle to understand what he just went through), shame (over his actions), grief (from the reaction of his loved ones), and fear (that he will act that way again). In short, he resembles a closed-off war veteran suffering from post traumatic stress disorder.

But this inhibited state does not last. Soon the child's control slips and he re-enters that other state, forming disturbing visions, losing his inhibitions, and acting wild all over again. Inhibited is a good word to describe how you yourself feel around such children. You may even suspect that they are not truly introverted by nature, but are deliberately inhibiting themselves, perhaps hoping that by doing so they can gain better control over themselves, at least over their violent side.

Another possible scenario is that of a child whose predominant trait had been wildness, but after a period of time the wildness left. Now you see him becoming increasingly introverted, not able to understand his previous behavior yet not quite able to let go of it. At this point they have moved in a slow progression from the predominantly overreacting segment to the predominantly closing off segment.

I would like to make one last point in relation to introversion. Once a *Stramonium* child stops being *Stramonium*, either because he has received the remedy or has left that layer for some other reason, he may be unprepared for the world that he will face. Having been wild for a period of time, the child may now realize, for the first time, that his parents no longer treat him with the loving care that they used to. While he was in the *Stramonium* state, he took all that the parents had. They are now spent. At this point, you will find some of them being harsh or even abusing their child, while others maintain a cool stance as 'concerned' parents.

The sheer loneliness that the child lives in at this time, may make him extremely sad. It is at this juncture, as he experiences his lonely life and grief, that he enters a *Natrum muriaticum* or *Staphysagria* state. I consider these two remedies to be complementary to *Stramonium*. I strongly advise the family to undertake counseling at this point. Now that the child has left the violent layer behind, the parents must too leave behind their bad feelings and start anew to reconstruct a loving, mutually nurturing relationship.

This may indeed be very difficult for the parents to do, but it is crucial that they do so during this critical transition from that dark world the child was living in to the world we inhabit.

## Depression

Though it is not often mentioned in the literature, *Stramonium* can easily enter into intense depression. There are actually two manifestations of this depression, one that is nearer to the violent segment of the *Stramonium* cycle, the other nearer to the shut down/dead segment.

The first type may occur either in the midst of a tumultuous fit or following rage or it may occur during an excessive period of aggression or violence, when the child is experiencing repercussions from his actions. He can get so frustrated that he may say he wants to kill himself.

Ten year old Monroe is a good example of this first type. His family is accustomed to depression. His grandfather and uncle had both committed suicide, and other people in the family were in treatment for depression and manic depression. Because Monroe loved his parents and also feared being separated from them, when he started kindergarten he already had begun showing signs of depression. As soon as his mother dropped him off at school he would throw himself on the ground, kicking and punching himself and crying, "I hate myself." These temper tantrums and fits only grew worse over the succeeding years. Whenever he made a mistake or felt an increase of stress, he would stiffen up, grit his teeth, and begin to hit himself, saying, "I'm stupid. I want to die. It's all my fault." He took to being a recluse, sticking to himself, making no friends. Whenever his parents had to go somewhere, leaving him for an evening or a whole day, he would revert to these same statements about wishing for death or intending to hurt himself.

Just as other children fantasize, so did Monroe. But while their fantasies were pleasant or adventuresome, his were nightmarish fantasies about killing or being killed. The combination of self-inflicted violence, strong fears, and a forsaken feeling led to a prescription of *Stramonium*, which was curative.

This example so closely resembles examples in the **Violence** section that it may be mistaken for yet another expression of the violent or destructive segment. It is true that this type of violence does look familiar, but the main

## THE ELEMENT OF CLOSING OFF; INTROVERSION

difference here is that the self loathing and depression cause the child to close off and turn the violence inward where it takes its toll within him and upon him. While the impulse to suicide in these cases is closer to a fit of anger than to morose depression, the children who behave in this manner are clearly on their way to a long term depression. This type of depression looks a lot like *Medorrhinum* with its fitful anger that alternates with depression and feelings of suicide.

The second kind of depression is more closely associated with the introverted and shut down/dead segment of *Stramonium*. At this point the child may be past the 'acting out' type of depression and grown increasingly introverted and depressed. Now he begins to live like a recluse, spending more and more time alone. His mildness is built out of an inferiority complex, thinking morbid thoughts, as before, but now the morbidity turns to thoughts of how to hurt himself. It is at this time that *Stramonium* may fantasize about cutting himself with a razor or killing himself outright. He may find this life too hard and may actually believe that he is causing too much trouble in the family and that it will be easier on everyone if he just ends his life.

Often the depression will be seen accompanied by other segments of *Stramonium*, thus making the choice of the remedy easier. The fear, for instance, may still be present. And even if the violence has disappeared by this point, images of violence may remain. The movies he chooses to watch will most likely be ones that contain violence. His dreams will probably be violent as well. Even his stories or poems will have violent motifs.

Reclusive, depressed, filled with morbid and violent thoughts and fear, he now turns all the anguish inward, making severe depression or suicide a possible outcome. This kind of patient may be hard to distinguish from a severely depressed *Natrum muriaticum* at this point. But in *Stramonium* there is no self importance, no relishing the state as is found in *Natrum muriaticum*. This is not "I am miserable and loving it." It is real and self contained. This child is locked in a battle with darkness, gripped by anguish, agonizing over whether life is worth living. This is a serious state, a severe state, and should be treated as such.

# *The Element of Autism*

The fear and isolation felt by children (especially autistic children) stuck in this shut down/dead segment often elicit an anguished love in parents, care givers, and homeopaths. The agony of this aloneness can be felt in T.S. Eliot's words:

> Descend lower, descend only
> Into the world of perpetual solitude,
> World not world, but that which is not world,
> Internal darkness, deprivation
> And destitution of all property,
> Desiccation of the world of sense,
> Evacuation of the world of fancy,
> Inoperancy of the world of spirit;
> This is the one way, and the other
> Is the same, not in movement
> But abstention from movement; while the world moves
> In appetency, on its metalled ways
> Of time past and time future.
> from *Four Quartets*

*Stramonium* is a remedy commonly used in the treatment of autistic children. Although autism is generally a difficult problem to treat, I have found that homeopathic treatment can often bring about positive changes, with the child becoming less aggressive, less self-stimulating, less ritualistic and more communicative. Sometimes a miracle happens. The child comes back to us and is once again able to express himself verbally. Though I have used a number of remedies in the treatment of autism, here I will only be describing that autism which has responded well to *Stramonium*.

Perhaps an analogy would be helpful in presenting a picture of the symptoms of the autistic *Stramonium* child, as they appear in the shut down segment of the remedy, the death element. What do you suppose would happen to you if someone took you, altered your perceptions to flood you with fears, put you in a coffin, and buried you alive?

Terror. Sheer unfathomable terror is what most of us would feel. That is exactly the state the *Stramonium* child enters into. And in that state, every terrifying image of the dark side of life, every semblance of evil, springs to life. Absolute terror grips him. Evil is no longer merely a word or a feeling, but rather a milieu that engulfs him. He feels as if tainted by the touch of some unclean hand that will ultimately ravage him. In that terror, in that darkness, the *Stramonium* child comes to realize an alarming truth—that we are born alone and die alone. And this discovery gives birth to a profound sense of isolation.

One of the effects of all this terror is that the child becomes plagued by images of horror and death. Some *Stramonium* patients have described this existence as "living in hell", and after a while they can no longer differentiate the behaviors of that life from acceptable behaviors. They do not even realize that they are acting out the violence of that hell.

To try to protect himself from this terrifying hell, the child may begin to psychically fold into himself. And so autism becomes a type of protective mechanism for him, a way of hiding. Also possible is that the child, stuck in a world full of monstrous visions, becomes entranced or psychically paralyzed by his terror and can no longer work his way back into this world. This paralysis is perhaps what brings on the autistic traits that are so commonly seen in this remedy. Both examples show how wanting to close off can overshoot into shutting down too much.

Before further describing the autism, I would like to clarify three points. First of all, the analogies of hell and being buried that are used in this section are not my invention. They are the very words used by these children and young adults when describing the lesser states of autism. Even the parents use such language in telling us what they notice about their children. Truly, this is exactly what one feels from these children while observing them.

Secondly, some *Stramonium* children are in fact autistic, while others only have autistic traits, such as ritualism or self-abusive behavior. In addition, there are those who appear to be autistic, but actually have temporal lobe epilepsy, Landau-Kleffner syndrome, or other neurologic problems.

Thirdly, once parents become aware of what the *Stramonium* state involves, they may begin to accept that the child simply cannot keep himself from his violent actions or outrageous behaviors. Understanding this may help to mollify the feelings of frustration or anger experienced daily by the parent. The parents or siblings of such a child should be forewarned that if they act in a way that might be seen by the child as threatening, the syndrome will, without question, become more difficult to treat. On the other hand, if they strive to provide the *Stramonium* child with a very safe environment, his autistic traits will not develop as quickly or as deeply.

**Autistic Traits**

The reasons why some children come into the world in an infolded autistic *Stramonium* state will vary, but one of the most common causes is fright, perhaps a severe fright the mother experienced during pregnancy. The mother might say, "I wonder why I can't get over that scary character in the movie," not realizing that the fetus may have experienced the fright as well, and that the excessive and prolonged reaction she is experiencing is due to the baby and not to her. Later, the baby is born and displays certain autistic traits.

It is also possible that a baby's initial fright came from the feeling that occurred when the umbilical cord was wrapped around the neck or from being stuck and trapped in the birth canal. After such an experience, when the baby is born, he may have a vacant look and seem uninterested in his surroundings. From that point on the baby begins to show autistic traits.

Another parent describes how the infolding behaviors developed little by little. Brianna says of her three year old daughter, "Probably every parent thinks this, but she seemed so bright. She had a shine and sparkle in her eyes and would follow everything that was said in the room. But ever since Halloween when her brother scared her with his mask, she just seems to isolate herself more and more. I mean she kind of looks dumb. She goes off by herself and doesn't play with the other kids like she used to. Now she only wants to play solitary games. She sits at the kitchen table and tries to draw or watercolor, and her head rolls from side to side. We call to her but she doesn't hear us. We have to come around and pull her away from what she's doing before she'll come back to the family."

Another mother attributes the infolding to a feeling of being forsaken.

# STRAMONIUM

"After his father and I broke up, little Bill cut himself off from everything and chose to be in his own world. He became so elusive. If he doesn't like someone or dislikes the surroundings, he disappears within himself."

There are a number of possible scenarios that may contribute to altering a child's perceptions. It could happen due to some injury to the brain, be it from trauma or infection or even as a reaction to a vaccination. For example, a child may have been born absolutely normal, but after a specific event, such as an infection, the autistic symptoms of *Stramonium* begin to appear. One father said, "Since the bronchitis, Steve won't listen to me any more. My wife says he seems to be happy enough just looming in his own world."

Another father, another child—this time the autism started after a bad influenza. "He used to be so sweet, but now he's a handful." Joe, who is two, yells and jabbers loudly, rocking fast and hard on his rocking chair, his mother holding him down. Watching his frenetic energy, I feel a wild imagination in a wild child in a wild world—all inside his head. A child like this, trapped in a world filled with violence, is not even aware that he is acting in a bizarre manner. He stares into space and seems oblivious to our presence. His father confirms this. "He does not come out and share what he is experiencing."

The mother picks up the thread of conversation, "Until he got a really bad flu seven months ago, he used to sit up and talk and actually had four and five word sentences. But since then, each day he becomes more and more like this." The mother has to shake him to focus, otherwise he has a glazed look, staring at the space in front of him, his eyes glistening and wide open. When he does manage to focus, his actions are more in keeping with those of this world, though they are still those of a hyperactive child, tossing books and toys all over the floor.

## Ritual / Perseverative Behavior

One common aspect of autism is ritualistic behavior. In *Stramonium*, this behavior can be adopted for different reasons. The most common seems to be as a way to allay fears, anxieties, and as a way to control himself. If the ritual is broken, this type of child becomes frightened and uncontrollable. After all, a fairly common strategy for dealing with fears is that of over-control, and over-control, when taken to extremes, leads to shutting down, to ritualistic behaviors. "If Alexandria finds herself in any situation that is uneasy

# THE ELEMENT OF AUTISM

for her, she always reacts the same way. First she climbs on my lap, and wants me to hug her. Then I have to place my right hand over my left (usually I hold her with the left over the right). If I fail to do it that certain way, she will begin to scream and take it out on me. Once we have gone through our routine and she feels safe, she will say blankly, 'Put me down,' as if I am not needed any more. It's almost as if we felt no connection in the hug, or maybe it's just that the emotion doesn't seem to last beyond the time she gets over her fear."

A second reason relates to the trance-like state. This type of child walks about as though unconscious, seemingly unaware of life. In this state of unawareness, he cannot think or be spontaneous, and so he falls into ritually doing the same thing over and over.

A third reason for the ritualistic behavior is the need to control others and/or instill fear in them. As Niccolo Machiavelli wrote in *The Prince*, "Since love and fear can hardly exist together, if we must choose between them, it is far safer to be feared than loved." This kind of child, similar to the *Lycopodium* child, becomes ritualistic to gain control. When things do not go as he wishes, he will misbehave, becoming unruly and violent.

So, even in the realm of ritual we find the two sides of *Stramonium*. On the one hand there is the side that wants to live and uses ritual to allay fears and protect himself; on the other hand there is the dark side that uses violent rituals to threaten and frighten others and thus control them.

Andrew's story shows the multipurpose of ritual in *Stramonium*. As a result of a severely traumatic birth, Andrew experienced moderate physical developmental delays, similar to those of a mild cerebral palsy. Because of this, he was isolated from the other children, which in turn created an emotional delay. He began to develop many fears, including witches, dogs, and any noise that was not immediately explainable. As the fears mounted Andrew produced another side to his personality. He became obstinate, fighting with his parents both physically and verbally. As his fearfulness and aggressiveness increased, he also began to develop obsessions and rituals involving his dress, his food, his room, and his toys. If anything went contrary to his expectations (that is, contrary to the way it had always gone), he would first exhibit fright and then shift automatically into a violent mode. So, here again we find ritual leading to fear then to violence and back to the ritual element once more.

# STRAMONIUM

Perseverating may also be seen in an autistic *Stramonium* child's eating or drinking habits. One mother describes her son's patterns. "If Stan wants something to drink, I give it to him, but then he hurls the cup and throws a temper tantrum, something I have grown accustomed to. It might take up to twenty minutes to understand that yes he was thirsty, but no it was not the cup he wanted. He has become so easily frustrated, so brittle. I have to prepare food for him in a certain way, each time, in order for us to have a semblance of a calm meal. He hates mixed up foods. If the foods on the plate touch each other, or if they are mixed up as in a casserole, he begins to fuss, and if we do not catch it right at that moment, he will throw the dish on the floor. He'll have a temper tantrum if I say, 'So long son,' because I'm supposed to say, 'Bye-bye baby.' When he was just five years old I would watch him go up the stairs only to come back down, so he could go up 'properly' (or what's proper to him). The opposite foot had to be on the stairs exactly the way it has always been before."

Another mother describes her concerns. "Alan has become very ritualistic about some ordinary aspects of his day. I'll watch him run down the steps at school, stop himself, cry, and say, 'I didn't do it right,' then retrace his steps and descend over and over again, adding some step he left out before. On the drive home he insists that I say, 'Yes' to the same questions he asks at the same place, the same time. Every drive home, every day, I have to go through this. He also has taken to watching me do things, and if he feels he has missed something or misunderstood something, he screams and cries, and we have to do it all over again."

Another child developed a different version on ritual behavior. "Roberto began his perseverative obsessions very early in his life, but his fifth year was the big watershed year. He got stuck on different interests. One time it was guns and swords. He cut knives and guns out of cardboard and hid them all over his room. He talked about them constantly, drew them, cut pictures of them out of magazines and newspapers and spent most of his museum time in the weapons room. On first meeting Roberto, people think it's cute, you know, the way kids get into stuff for a while. But before long they see how totally obsessed he is and become uncomfortable around him."

In addition to the more commonly seen autistic traits mentioned already, such as an infant who makes no eye contact, there are less troublesome traits associated with autism that illustrate the ritual nature. "Margie loves smells and colors. She has become finicky about what she is going to eat or play with. She will only tolerate certain things. Above all else, whatever she handles must have an agreeable smell. We don't know what that means, you know, how she makes the decision. But she will smell a toy and decide whether to play with it or not. I mean, she's smelling plastic."

There are also children who are disturbed to a lesser degree. One such child has a healthy sense of aesthetics but plays by herself in a world of her own invention. "Mary plays with bright colored toys and likes to smell flowers and toys. She has a great imagination. But everything she plays with, even the Legos, are always sailing ships." It turns out that this is a child whose mother became petrified after being out in a boat on a windy sea.

After her child took the remedy, another mother tells me, "I can see Sue coming out of her shell. She has learned some skills, is not so afraid, and is aware of other children for the first time in ages. She likes to play with us (the family) and likes to play with other children in play-group now."

## Fastidiousness

In addition, there are children whose tendency toward autistic or ritualistic behavior can be seen in their fastidiousness. Not well known for this remedy, and yet fairly commonly found in a subset of children and adults, is a strong desire for cleanliness. It may be noted as early as age one in a child who is so picky that he cannot stand to have gooey or sticky fingers and will demand that they be wiped after eating. Or you may see it in the two year old who picks up after himself and tidies up the mess he left on the floor, or in the teenager who cleans her room without being asked and keeps rearranging the furniture or insists on wearing particularly clean clothes.

While this point should be highlighted, since it is not well known for the remedy, it is also necessary to differentiate it from other remedies that have this fastidiousness. It is not the cleanliness itself that is the focus, but rather its meaning in relation to the rest of the picture. In a child who is surrounded by a world that is monstrous, dark, and grotesque, it is not a wonder if he compensates by becoming very neat. It is one way of trying to find a balance, but then it overshoots and becomes a problem. The other thing that motivates this desire for cleanliness is the ritualistic driven side of the child. So we can say it is not so much that they are intent on the cleanliness as that their obsessiveness and rigidity drive them to these perseverative behaviors which make them strive for precision and clarity. They want things black and white. In cases like this, a child may develop the same conscientiousness for trifles that is usually only seen in adults. And so being rigid, closed, or unchanging in any form fits into this segment.

**Full Autism**

There are several fully described subtypes of autistic syndromes. Two that seem to appear often at the homeopath's office are: pervasive developmental delay (or a full autistic trait) and Landau-Kleffner syndrome.

The *Stramonium* child with fully autistic/pervasive developmental disorder may begin life like many other children. However, there may be a question about the hearing ability, as these children are prone to repeated otitis medias and often are on antibiotics and/or may have tubes in the ears. And even though they may be contented, happy, and affectionate most of the time, they tend to ultimately develop an intense fear of the dark, of closed rooms, and of being bathed. In these situations they will shriek and scream. The parents often report being up with this screaming child at night, walking him to try to lessen the fear or ease the pain of an earache or colic. As these children approach two or two and a half, they still may not speak, or may have the sensory/motor development of a one year old, or at three years may show no desire to be toilet trained. They may develop tactile defensiveness, keeping their fingers separated, not touching objects, or alternately liking to play in sand or shaving cream. These children may not show the full *Stramonium* picture—the violence may be lacking—yet the rest of the picture will fit the remedy. Thus we can observe a progression in this illness: infections that expose the child to pain and then to fear of pain, inflammations/overreactions leading to closing off and fear; infections which in turn lead to altered perceptions that give birth to horrors, after which an infolding of the personality begins, moving him once again toward aggressive behavior.

In the office you see this child walking back and forth, touching one object after another, but usually not with the intense restlessness of autistic children who need other remedies than *Stramonium*. The restlessness, for me, is an important clue, for the primary issue in the *Stramonium* autistic child will not usually be hyperactivity. Rather, the outstanding impression will be that of a child stuck in a world of his own, a world filled with a violence just waiting to be unleashed. But if, in the child's presence, you feel a whirlwind of energy seeking an outlet, then you will do well to look at several other remedies, such as *Veratrum album*, *Tarentula hispanica* or *Lachesis*.

One of the most interesting subtypes of autism that I have encountered is Landau-Kleffner syndrome. It usually begins around age three but has been known to start as late as six. It affects children who start out as normal or above average bright children, and then all of a sudden they begin to lose their ability to understand speech or to communicate. The child is aware of the deterioration in his communication skills but is unable to stop it. There are often EEG changes corresponding to the temporal lobe and sometimes there will be seizures. The children who retain the ability to communicate will often do so in a forced staccato telegraphic speech. Different children deal with this change in different ways. Some of them can understand their problem and will compensate by developing good writing skills or even sign language. They are, for the most part, above average in intelligence and score quite high on IQ tests.

In others, the diminished ability to speak can lead to altered perceptions and from there to drastic changes in behavior. Some of these children develop ritualistic self stimulating behaviors. It is these children that may benefit from *Stramonium*. They may become unpredictably violent, and, like *Hyoscyamus*, may all of a sudden begin to destroy objects or even attempt to kill. They may also develop fears at night accompanied by seizures. Sometimes they become perfectionistic, throwing temper tantrums if the parent does not say or do (to perfection) exactly what they wish. In addition, these children may become hyperactive. While several remedies might be considered for them, *Stramonium* is high on the list.

As a child's lack of ability to understand the verbal world grows, he becomes frustrated by his loss of control over the conscious mind and more and more isolated and fearful about what is happening to him. Once again, in these disordered children, you can see the same progression: the inability to speak somehow leads to altered perceptions and then to frustrations, fears, an infolding of the psyche and retreat from this world, and finally to a full *Stramonium* picture—the reign of the unconscious, which transforms the child into a terror.

# STRAMONIUM

The thing about Landau-Kleffner syndrome that is so interesting to me is that a child who was average or above average linguistically, all of a sudden has that part of him cut off, and yet he retains his intelligence. It has been fascinating listening to these children describe the process of losing their speech and then gaining it back again. In this in-between world, they form a sort of middle ground between us and the autistic children that do not communicate at all. This is reminiscent of the state explored in the night terror portion of the *Sleep* section, a state in which, also, the child is trapped between the fully conscious mind and the mind that is stuck in a sleep stage.

Out of the war raging within *Stramonium*, an orphan is created. Alone, forsaken, exposed to the elements—the contradictions inside himself are too great to bear. He enters the battle already scarred. The battle continues and the behaviors begin. One of these behaviors is autism.

Often, after *Stramonium* has begun to do its work, words will begin to come out of the child, and soon after that, short sentences may appear. Really, a miracle occurs. Some children make fantastic progress in a short period of time, communicating again and even growing emotionally. Other children just manage to make better contact. They seem more aware of what is expected of them, but their delay continues. Instead of being behind by three years they may now be behind by only two, but they are still behind.

Unfortunately, it is not possible for us to tell just how much a child will improve after a remedy is given. I had once believed that the more severe the condition was, the less likely a great outcome would be achieved. But I have been surprised by these miracles. On the other hand, I have treated children who were only moderately affected, and while the results were gratifying to all, I was still not quite satisfied. I could not help but think that there should have been more improvement. But miracles do happen, sometimes with the help of *Stramonium*.

# *Sleep*

> ...at that more truthful hour when my eyes closed to the things of the outer world (on whose frontier intellect and will, momentarily paralyzed, could no longer strive to rescue me from the cruelty of my real impressions) reflected, refracted the agonizing annihilation, in the mysteriously lighted darkness of my organs. World of sleep in which our inner consciousness placed in bondage to the disturbances of our organs, quickens the rhythm of heart and breath because a similar dose of terror, sorrow, remorse, acts with a strength magnified a hundredfold if it is thus injected into our veins; as soon as, to traverse the arteries of the subterranean city, we have embarked upon an inward Lethe meandering sixfold, huge solemn forms appear to us, approach, and glide away, leaving us in tears.
>
> Proust, from *Sodomme et Gomorrhe* 22-224

Along with the mental-emotional realm and the nervous system, the realm of sleep offers the most insight into the *Stramonium* cycle. In fact this area is so rich in confirmatory symptoms that **if you have a child with absolutely no sleep symptoms to verify a prescription of *Stramonium*, it is unlikely to be the correct remedy.**

That there are so many sleep symptoms is not surprising, for it is during sleep and in the process of drifting off to sleep, that the conscious mind finally relinquishes control and the unconscious mind takes over. It is here, in the night, that everything held in check during the day will finally be expressed. The intense battle-line between conscious and unconscious, so carefully drawn throughout the day, shifts during the night, as one side loses its ability to fight and the other gains in power. As the images of death increase, the segments having to do with stillness, with death, grow stronger, and this serves to intensify the segment of fear in the child.

# STRAMONIUM

This battle can be witnessed in three different areas. **The presence of symptoms in any one of these areas can be used to confirm the need for *Stramonium:***

- Fears before Sleep
- Nightmares and Night Terrors
- General Sleep Symptoms

Each of these categories will be presented separately, but first I would like to draw the reader's attention to a valuable book for understanding children's sleep, Richard Ferber's *Solve Your Child's Sleep Problems*, published by Simon and Schuster. This book is most helpful in developing a fuller understanding of sleep cycles and sleep disturbances. I strongly recommend chapters one, four, and five for parents and clinicians alike.

## Fears Before Sleep

**Fear of going to bed** is a fairly characteristic symptom found in most *Stramonium* children. Many young children will be unable to voice specific reasons for their fears, but older children will commonly admit to: **fear of the dark, of monsters, of being left alone,** and such fears as are often associated with **movies and stories recently seen or heard.** A more common cause for bedtime fears, whether the child verbalizes it or not, is a previous history of terrifying dreams. It is the **terror of repeating such dreams** that makes a *Stramonium* child fear going to sleep. One gets the feeling that there is a battle raging within the child between a dark demonic side and the forces of light. Each night, there surfaces within the child an overwhelming sense that, at some deep level, he is about to go through those same horrible visions—visions of torture, of terror. And so, each night, he resists his parents' attempts to put him to bed, and even more desperately resists falling asleep.

Many authorities on sleep disorders believe that nighttime fears are brought about by some stress or anxiety that has occurred during the day but only surfaces at night. The stresses may be *external* in origin, such as fear of being separated from the mother or the kind of fears that often accompany a divorce. There may also exist a justifiable fear of being beaten or violated in some way, which can develop after the child has been abused. Even one beating can bring on such fear.

# SLEEP

Stresses may also be *internal* in origin. At the time when the child is developing impulse control, when he wants to misbehave, his impulsive side may begin to struggle with and fight against his controlling side. Most children ultimately work this out, but the *Stramonium* child does not. In observing the child's attempts to establish control over impulses, the parent or practitioner will witness the following sequence unfolding in an introverted *Stramonium* child: first, he feels a strong impulse to misbehave (the violent overreaction segment), then guilt over this impulse mounts (the closing off/introversion segment), so he struggles to control it, which makes him hypervigilant and anxious about relinquishing control (the shut down/ dead segment). No wonder he becomes increasingly more fearful of going to bed and has so much trouble falling asleep. He worries and worries, although quite unable to pinpoint why he is worried in the first place. In truth, he is worrying about his own impulses. **The darkness or monsters that these children fear are nothing more than their own impulses buried deep in the unconscious.** The horrible nightmares and night terrors spring out from these buried impulses. Herman Melville expressed this well in *Pierre*, "One trembles to think of that mysterious thing in the soul, which seems to acknowledge no human jurisdiction, but in spite of the individual's own innocent self, will still dream horrid dreams and mutter unmentionable thoughts."

In the *Stramonium* child you are likely to see certain typical behaviors at bedtime. Many of these, in one way or another, exemplify the rubric: **MIND: Clinging.** During the preverbal stage, from eight to fifteen months, the child may scream when being put to bed. No matter how hard a mother may try to ensure a smooth, love-filled transition from the waking state into the sleep state, the outcome is more likely to be such loud shrieking that it renders her temporarily deaf. Despite continued attempts on her part to soothe the child, he will shut his eyes tight and scream at the top of his lungs. This bedtime shrieking often resembles that of *Medorrhinum, Tuberculinum, Lycopodium, Chamomilla, Borax, Cina* or *Calcarea phosphorica*. All the mother's warm, soothing words and the loving tone of voice do not penetrate through whatever horrible thing it is that envelops the child at that time.

So every night a push/pull scenario takes place. When picked up, the little one will struggle and resist and pull away, which only exasperates the parent. At the very same time he may be asking to sleep in the parents' bed, where he sleeps best, especially if actually in contact with the parent. Sometimes he will be content if the parent lies down with him in his bed, but as he drifts off, as soon as the parent attempts to rise quietly and tiptoe away, the child will startle, half-awake, and begin to cry anew.

An older child will be more likely to express his fear of going to sleep by acting out or by strongly resisting any request made throughout the evening that even hints of bedtime. A simple suggestion such as, "Time to brush your teeth," will set the child off like a time-bomb. The parents begin to wonder if their child is crazy. The therapist may describe him as irrational, impulsive, or oppositional. Yet, in reality, the child is scared witless but lacks the verbal maturity required to express it. Often the parent, failing to realize what's behind this irritating and confusing behavior, tries to force the child to go to sleep. But because he is unable to express what is bothering him, he resists, and a major conflict follows. These bedtime wars only further disrupt the already shaky parent/child relationship.

Unfortunately, the battle waged between parent and child over the terrain of the *Stramonium's* psyche never engages the real enemy (the fear, the isolation, the confusion). Moreover, the conflict only seems to deepen the child's pain, causing a further expansion of the breach in the containment of his unconscious, which results in his spiraling even deeper within the same cycle. **The *Stramonium* child experiences these injunctions and actions (such as forcing him to go to bed) as attempts to alienate or isolate him. Even worse, he feels abandoned to his fate—a night full of hideous visions.**

**To deal with these fears, the child may develop an almost opposite strategy to the time-bomb behavior, a strategy of over-control.** He may begin to act rigidly, even exhibit **ritualistic behaviors**. One parent described her daughter's bedtime ritual. "She insists that I read the same book every night. Then I have to rub her back clockwise for a while, then counter-clockwise. Then she turns, sighs, and says, 'Go,' dismissing me with a word, as if my services are no longer required."

If the child is older, he may be able to articulate his nighttime fears, citing specific events from the past that frightened him. Some children report frights from experiences such as being attacked by a person or an animal. They become increasingly upset by the possibility of this fright recurring as night closes in. Most commonly in contemporary North

## SLEEP

America, the fears mentioned will stem from **violence seen on television or in the movies. Seeing such violence heightens a child's sense of insecurity in the world, thus creating the etiology that will make the child's cycle spiral deeper and deeper, creating worse symptoms.**

As mentioned in the *Mind: Fear* section, the *Stramonium* child has a **strong fear of the dark.** This is expressed most vehemently at night, often in the form of an intense fear of being **abandoned and alone in the dark.** Parents may take to leaving a light on so the child can derive comfort from it. As George Vithoulkas noted, even after the *Stramonium* child is asleep, if you turn off the light, the child will wake up at once and scream. Many other remedy-types will not be awakened at all by a suddenly darkened room.

There are very specific **modalities** to look for in *Stramonium* regarding fears. They are **worse** from watching a **scary movie,** hearing **a scary story,** or taking a **shower or bath** in the evening. **Sleeping alone in a dark room also serves to intensify the fears.**

The child feels **better** from **sleeping with the light on and/or sleeping with the parent** to whom he feels most bonded. But, in my experience, it is not advisable to encourage the *Stramonium* child who is experiencing nighttime fears to sleep in the parents' bed. With this type of child, the 'family bed' arrangement may work for a while, but eventually it backfires. The contact with his parents may temporarily soothe the child, but, as the parents bemoan, it tends to increase his dependence on them. The child senses that this cannot last forever and that eventually he will be once again abandoned and alone in his own room. This only increases his fears. Another disadvantage to this arrangement is that after several months the child may even replace one of the parents, as the bed is no longer big enough for the three of them—certainly not the outcome originally intended.

There are things that can be done to help him overcome his fears. Many psychologists suggest that it is important that the child spend as much quality time as possible in his own bedroom during the daytime hours. Playing there often, or having a parent read to him there, will encourage him to feel secure in his own room, until it becomes a safe haven for him, a place where he knows he can let his guard down. Regarding fear of a darkened room, I often advise parents to leave a light on somewhere, so it will stream into the room. Most children sleep better with some light on. Then if they do awake at night, there is enough light for them to orient themselves.

# STRAMONIUM

## Nightmares and Night Terrors

> The dream is the small hidden door in the deepest and most intimate sanctum of the soul, which opens into that primeval cosmic night that was soul long before there was a conscious ego and will be soul far beyond what a conscious ego could ever reach.
>
> from Carl Gustav Jung's
> *The Meaning of Psychology for Modern Man*

I would like to stress for parent and practitioner alike that, while the whole of the *Sleep* section offers information that is of special importance in recognizing *Stramonium*, the section on night terrors is even more revealing. In conversation with physicians and parents I have found that many have not yet formed a clear understanding of nightmares and night terrors or other sleep disturbances. If parents can come to an awareness of the process that is involved, they may be able to do things that will break the pattern of their child's night terrors and the behavior problems that result from them. Further, if a cycle of abuse and punishment has developed in dealing with the night terrors, the parent will be better able to halt it or at least wind down from it.

Giving the child the correct remedy is certainly of prime importance in breaking the cycle. But there are also certain techniques that many parents have found beneficial. I hope that the following discussion of nightmares and night terrors will help parents to help their child successfully overcome his problems.

A **nightmare** is a very scary dream that occurs *during REM sleep*. In most children, nightmares tend to occur when the child has been undergoing emotional stress or has experienced a fright during the day similar to the fears they express at bedtime, such as fear of ghosts or dogs. It is not the nightmare itself that is the problem but rather the stresses that the child undergoes during the day. The nightmare serves to mirror those stresses.

The child's tense vigilance at night, due to fears, comes to color his dreams, causing frightening images to appear. But when he wakes, the difference between dream and reality is not clear to him (the confusion segment). This terrifies him, so he hunts for his parents, seeking consolation and protection. It is extremely important that they give him this consolation and reassure him that he is safe.

## SLEEP

The nightmares of *Stramonium* involve **harm** and **being hurt, threats, animals, and images from scary movies.** The following are typical of children's nightmares: Alan screams, "Some animals are in my room!" Lynne, weeping, cries out, "A shark came out of the water! It's eating my family!" Harry shouts, "Wolves are after me! They're going to kill me!" Duane yells out in his sleep, "A dog is chasing me!" Jerry is sure that, "A horrible monster is coming up out of the water and it's looking for me." Bruce tells me, "I heard a ghost story a year ago, and I still can't get it out of my head. I keep dreaming about it. That's what my nightmare is always about. It always ends the same way, with these nails digging into my eyes."

More dramatic even than nightmares, however, are **night terrors.** *It is vital to understand two points about the night terror. First of all, night terrors are not within the child's control or will. Secondly, yelling, hitting, or in any way punishing the child will hurt rather than help the child. Further, it will increase the night terror episodes, either in frequency or in duration.*

Night terrors are experiences which occur *during partial waking from deep sleep.* The child is emerging from one of the most profound stages of sleep, the non-REM stage, in which he has spent an hour to an hour and a half, and it is at that time, when he suddenly changes to a lighter sleep stage, that the night terrors occur. Often they will be triggered by noise or a touch or a change of light. Even though the shift occurs abruptly, it usually is natural and uncomplicated, but not always for *Stramonium.* **In some of these children the transition is neither smooth nor short and may itself lead to a night terror.**

This is, in part, because the sleep of the very young is so deep (deeper than that of adults) that they may not be able to recognize the cue to change sleep states, so they remain partially in a deep sleep state, while at the same time partially entering a waking state. *According to Ferber, during that time, the night terror child is 'stuck' in between the two stages and simultaneously exhibits brain patterns and behaviors of both the sleep state and the waking state.* It is sort of like the state of an adult who is suddenly awakened by some emergency and needs to act immediately, but finds that his actions and thinking are confused for a period of seconds or even minutes. A child's confusion in one of these night terrors can last anywhere from a few minutes up to an hour. This state of confusion, which results from being in two different states, is typical of the confusion segment of the cycle and soon leads the child into the segment of fear.

# STRAMONIUM

Stuck between the sleep and waking states, the child behaves as if in danger. His words and actions indicate that he is trying to escape from something or keep something at bay. He is, in fact, stuck between two states. As he makes the transition from partial sleep into partial awakening, the *Stramonium* child, in all probability, is experiencing a flood of all the fears, anxieties and terrors which had been lying low in the unconscious, but which are now emerging to color all that his senses are exposed to. Thus, a light may be perceived as a fire, a parent as a monster, a picture as a ghost. An ordinary noise may sound like a wild animal to him. And so he thrashes about in terror, trying to escape from these frightening images. The rubrics that illustrate these behaviors are: **MIND: Escape, attempts to; MIND: Fear;** and **MIND: Delusion, of being injured.**

As we saw in the ***Stramonium Cycle*** section, the struggle between the unconscious and the conscious is a central concept in *Stramonium*. It is a tug of war between two states of reality, and it evokes both fear and confusion in the child. This duality is even more apparent in the sleep behaviors. Everything about night terrors points to *Stramonium* as the primary remedy to address these problems. *Calcarea carbonica* is the other most commonly needed remedy for night terrors in children.

Watching a child during a night terror is an unbelievably intense event. We cannot know exactly what the child experiences during the terror, because, since he remains partially asleep, he cannot answer our questions, and in the morning he does not even recall the event. The only clues we do have come from nightmares he has told us about, from which we extrapolate the content of the night terrors.

The following descriptions of *Stramonium* night terrors may help parents to identify them when they occur. John describes his son's night terrors: "All of a sudden he sits up and screams, with eyes wide open, looking right through me, yelling, 'It's eating my legs!' or 'Nnnoooo! Don't kill me!' or 'Aaaaghhhh! A big dog ate Jesse!' [his sister], or 'A wolf is chewing up my heart!'"

Laura and Peter tell a slightly different story. "James gets up screaming and wants us near because he's afraid to be alone in the dark. Mostly, he dreams that someone is killing one of us." Upon further examination, it is apparent that what these parents are calling dreams are really night terrors. "His eyes are closed and he's asleep during the whole episode.

## SLEEP

He gets out of bed and starts to punch the wall or tries to climb the curtain. He urinates on the floor, then walks all around the house, screaming the whole time. When we try to hold him, he pushes us away and kicks us or punches us, or sometimes he scratches us. When he's having these attacks, we have to shake him and slap him to try to snap him out of it. But he never wakes up, not even from being slapped. At some point he just falls asleep again, and then we put him in his bed and cover him up."

Alex describes a particular incident that occurred with his three year old, Michael: "We drove to a friend's house for supper. It took us about thirty minutes, and on the way there Michael fell asleep. I picked him up from the car and put him in the master bedroom with the lights on but pretty dim. Ten minutes later, I heard a slight noise coming from the room. I went in and saw him sitting up. I said, 'Hi, Mike.' He began to cry and squirm and thrash around. It got worse and worse. Nothing I tried seemed to make him happy. He just kept shrieking louder and louder. He screamed for his bottle, so I called to Alice, and she brought a juice bottle. But it wasn't his own bottle; it belonged to our host's baby, so he threw it down and shrieked even louder. At this point there was terror in his eyes. I tried to hug him but he pushed me away and scratched at me wildly, screaming and screeching. Finally I picked him up, even though he struggled and fought against me, and put him in the car. It was pretty dark outside. He panicked. He was thrashing and shrieking so loudly that it felt to me like his soul and body were being ripped apart. And then suddenly he stopped, looked around to figure out where he was, and calmly said something pleasant about the lights shining in a house we were driving past. It was over as suddenly as it had begun. He seemed not to be at all aware of what he had been through, though clearly he was wiped out. After another fifteen minutes of sighing and nodding, he fell asleep again. I cried myself to sleep that night."

Aaron describes his son Leo: "Nighttime used to be easy until Leo turned two. He started having the most intense dreams. Really frightening. He's lying there asleep, and all of a sudden I hear a noise from his bedroom. I look at the clock and it reads midnight. I go to Leo's room. He's moving his arm and moaning. Then he stops moving. About thirty seconds later, he yells out, 'Mommy! Mommy! No! No! No!' The whole time he's thrashing around, this way and that. He arches his body backwards. Sometimes his eyes are open and sometimes they're closed. He seems really scared, as if he is going to die. He thrashes around so much that he falls off the bed. Then the shock of that upsets him all the more. I want to help him, so I go to him and try to comfort him, but he starts to fight me. He acts terrified of me. He screams louder and thrashes some more. After a while he quiets down and eventually goes back to sleep. To tell you the truth, this is tearing at my heart. It's so painful watching your son go through hell and all you can do is stand by and watch. What am I doing wrong? Why is he going through this? Why can't I help him? I have never felt so powerless."

Ben, who is eight years old and a fraternal twin, had a nightmare that encompasses most of the *Stramonium* components: isolation, terror, death, being half alive, and the water element. Here is the dream: "I was in a city. It was weird and scary. There were weird sounds everywhere. I looked into a building and heard weird voices. Things moved that shouldn't. There were yucky swamps. And traps. Something would creep out and try to hit me if I went near, a spider web or something. My brother was with me. Weird statues all around. When I looked closely the statue turned older and older, yucky and wrinkled, like their bones showed, like someone had died. It was like a ghost land. A scary guy with a motorcycle came over to me and scared me. My big sister knew where to go to hide but I didn't, so I just huddled up. Then I went to a tree and it was spider-webby. I was walking on the sidewalk and the street was a swamp, very deep, and I didn't know what was in the water. I was scared the whole time, except when I was with my brother and sister. I'm always scared if I'm alone."

Night terrors are so dramatic and frightening to the onlooking parents that they often feel the need to do something in order to stop it; this at times aggravates the situation. For example, a scenario may begin by the parents tiptoeing quietly into the room and lovingly trying to cover the sleeping child better. The movement partially awakens the child and sends him into a night terror. The child screams and the scene quickly degenerates, at which point the parents may tell him to stop, but this only exacerbates the situation. Out of frustration, the parents finally start yelling. The look of panic grows worse on the child's face, but otherwise he does not respond, so the parents start shaking him, but he pulls away frantically, shrieking at the top of his voice.

At this point, if the family lives in an apartment, the neighbor comes upstairs to see what is the matter. Or if they live in a house, they are grateful

## SLEEP

that no one will hear the shrieking and think they are abusing their child. After several minutes of the screaming getting worse and worse, the parents may indeed wind up abusing their child. It begins with a light tap, then a slight shake, then a shove. By now the parents may get a little bit out of control and start yelling, "Stop it, stop it! Wake up, wake up!" as the night terror goes on and on. I know of people who have, at this point, thrown cold water on the child, in an attempt to awaken him. Not only do all these interventions not succeed, they actually aggravate the situation. Moreover, it is interesting to note how the *Stramonium* state in one person will cause a similar effect in the people around him. The mother who is watching her *Stramonium* child in this state will often experience a mixture of fright and violence herself, thus mirroring the fright and violence that the child feels and exhibits.

Advice as to what parents should do varies within the medical literature, according to the age of the child. If the child is young, most recommend that the parent sit close to him but not interfere with the night terror. Sitting nearby, the parent will be able to make sure the child does not hurt himself. Older children, however, may need different treatment. Their night terrors are often brought on by emotional stresses and over-control of their impulses. These children seem to do better when such conflicts and stresses are discussed openly so that, in time, they do not have to feel so guilty over their impulses that they resort to over-control.

*Guarding* is a term that Ferber uses for this over-control. Guarding, or vigilance, occurs when children experience so much anxiety that they cannot relax. They maintain this tension even in sleep and, when partially awakened, go straight into a night terror, just as a person facing a job interview may awaken anxiously in the night. In both instances, the daytime anxieties flow on through the sleeping state, and when the sleep becomes shallow, the sleeper gets caught in the undercurrent. However, what surfaces for the *Stramonium* child (similar to the adult's anxiety over a job interview) are those fears that remain submerged during the daytime hours, fears of devils, ghosts, and animals, or fears of abandonment and isolation.

While I agree with a great deal of the protocol regarding night terrors, I have found that with *Stramonium* children the strategy of waiting does not work well. These children do not seem to outgrow the night terror state. In fact, more often the opposite occurs: the child suffers more and more as each night he enters into the *Stramonium* state, and again and again his unconscious flows through and enlarges the breach into his conscious mind.

After listening to my patients and learning from them, I have tried a method over several years, which I believe is reliable, not only for communicating with the child and stopping the night terror, but also for eliminating the reasons why the night terrors occur in the first place. What I suggest to a parent depends on what I perceive to be the cause of that particular child's terror. (The constitutional state of the child, and the remedy needed, is of course always factored into any suggestions.) If the child is a *Stramonium*, and the traditional methods do not stop the night terrors, this method is well worth trying.

**This is essentially a four step process that can help to dispel or minimize night terrors. It aims:**

- to *identify* any stresses that might trigger the night terror
- to *diminish* the impact of that *stress by naming it*
- to *limit the frequency of exposure* to the stimuli
- to *open a passage* between the conscious and unconscious by naming the triggers.

For the *Stramonium* child, most of the triggers will relate to **such stresses as fear of abandonment or a fear of something evil that intends to injure them.** Therefore it is important for you, as a parent, to perceive exactly **which stresses trigger the night terrors.** For some children it will be a movie that frightened them, or simply washing their hair at night. For others swimming could be the stress that triggered the fear, or even a friendly dog that played nicely nearby that day. For still others, the stress could have been from the moment when mother disappeared around the corner of the house and, feeling alone, the toddler began to panic.

It is interesting that *Stramonium* **children will usually have night terrors if they urinate in their sleep,** although parents will rarely associate that with the night terror. The baby may urinate and feel the dampness and wake crying, or the toddler may urinate so much that he leaks through the diaper, wetting the bedclothes and mattress. This can happen also with older children when they wet the bed. In all these cases either it is the dampness that partially awakens the child or, conversely, it is upon entering a partially awakened state that the child urinates. I believe that the *Stramonium* child then interprets the urine as a bath, lake or some large body of water **(MIND: Fear, water, of)** and this triggers the night terror.

*The first step in eliminating the night terrors is to help the parents become aware of the different scenarios that are possible stresses for the child, for it is these that can trigger the night terrors. Knowing these stresses is a prerequisite to communicating with your terrified child during the night terror itself.* It is, after all, *powerlessness* that most parents say they feel as they watch their child in the grip of a night terror. As one parent put it, "Her eyes open in a horrific stare, as if she was about to meet the devil." Parents often express frustration at not knowing how to communicate with their child during a night terror or how to enter the child's domain and free him from his terror.

*The second step is to diminish the impact of the stress by talking about the fears or triggers before your child even gets into bed. During the evening, while he is busy doing something else, try to mention, casually or playfully, any event of the day that you think might have caused stress and might trigger a night terror.* By mentioning this trigger in passing, you may be able to dispel it. "That sure was a nice dog. Maybe it looked a little scary, but it was more like a puppy the way it rolled around and played with the ball and did anything you asked." And that is all! *Unless the child wants to talk about it, do not force the issue.* Accept that beyond airing the possibility, you must now wait for the child either to pick up the ball and run with it, or let it drop. (Take care not to build anything up larger than it is. By blowing something out of proportion, you could end up making the child even more anxious.) This second step accomplishes two objectives. First: It may decrease the night terrors if you validate daytime experiences that your child has had. Remember, you are modeling behavior for your child, as well as teaching him how to express emotion. Second: You will be putting in place, perhaps subliminally, a mechanism that your child can recognize later, in the half-sleep state.

*The third step is to decrease the frequency of exposure to any stimuli or stresses that seem to trigger the nightmares or night terrors.* For example, wash your child's hair in the morning rather than in the evening, thereby separating the event from his sleep by as much time as possible. Discourage video games and movies that are violent; they are inappropriate, at the very least, for this type of child. Also, take care that his bedroom is never in total darkness. These precautions will help to keep night terrors to a minimum.

## STRAMONIUM

Although they probably won't cure your child's night terrors, they will help to minimize their frequency in the near future. After the remedy has had enough time to act, *it alone* will often alleviate the problem. In time, these incidents will no longer be the triggers that they once were.

*The fourth step is to try to open a passageway between your child's conscious and unconscious states during the night terror by naming the things that might have triggered it. This step may be helpful for the child who still experiences night terrors after the beginning steps have already been established.* The parents still have powerful tools at their disposal, tools they developed through carrying out these first three steps. As mentioned earlier, one of the most frustrating things for many parents is their inability to communicate at the time of the night terror. *But with these tools you will be able to! Right in the middle of the night terror, you can come into the bedroom and, without restraining the child, begin to mention all the possible triggers for the night terror, triggers you know your child experienced that day or over the preceding few days. If this does not work, it might help to mention some trigger which your child tends to be sensitive to. If this also does not work, begin to mention your child's fears as these usually are the same as the triggers.* You will not have to go through a long list, for often the first or second word that you mention will turn out to be the relevant trigger. *Please do not just list these potential triggers. Work them into sentences, lovingly spoken in calm, reassuring tones.* If your child is in child care, it may be important to ask, at the end of each session, if anything happened during the day that may have scared him.

Whenever you mention the operative trigger, you may notice that your child, for the first time, makes a gesture that is different, or that he changes in some way. And you will realize that you are now finally able to contact your child while he is in the night terror state. One sign of such contact might be that his breathing deepens and he relaxes a few seconds after you mention the trigger word. For example, you might say something about water since you know that frightened the child. "Honey, it's okay. Are you dreaming about the shower? Do you think you're in the water again? You're not. You're in bed now, all dry and safe. You're just having a dream that you're in the water. Dad and Mom are here. We love you," and the breathing will change as he calms down. Or, "Are you dreaming about the dog? Do you think Fang is here? Don't be afraid. He's not here. He's not going to hurt you," and the eyes may lose that faraway stare as if beginning to see you for the first time, and he goes back to sleep. As you ask, "Is it the monster from the story? Are you seeing the guns from the movie?" you may see his face lose the grimace and his body lose its rigidity as he sinks into your arms.

As mentioned earlier, urinating in sleep can trigger a nightmare or night terror. This can happen even if the child is wearing a diaper that may have leaked, allowing him to become wet. He may not become fully awake but is just conscious enough to feel the discomfort of the wetness. Though current medical literature suggests that we not touch a child in the middle of a night terror, I differ with that opinion when the situation involves a wet *Stramonium* child. *The most essential thing is to make him dry again, by removing the pajamas or diaper, as well as changing the bedding. This will help ease his discomfort and shorten the night terror—as long as the parent does not have to pin the child down, thereby scaring him more and defeating the purpose.* At that time, hug your child protectively, soothingly, and murmuring loving, secure words about how you are there, how you will take care of him, assuring him that he is not alone, that it is only a dream about... (mention the fright), or telling him that he just urinated and is dry now, that he is safe, that the feared thing is not here in the room. This cascade of reassuring words, intermingled with the naming of his fears, will help him to believe you and feel trust in your presence. Frequently this will be enough to dispel the fear and end the night terror. Sometimes a child will wake up briefly, hear the careful naming of triggers and fears, and then go back to sleep. At other times, the child will simply relax and sleep easily in your arms as you talk to him and put him back down to sleep.

Why do I suggest this fourth step? Why should it work? Parents have often told me that, in the past, they have tried to hug their child and reassure him with kisses, but it has failed. Not only has he resisted them, but his distress was worsened by their tenderness. Why didn't hugging work before? Why may it work now? Because now there has been a link of communication established between parent and child. Now you can reach him where he is trapped—somewhere between a terrifying hell and the world he knows. It is the battle between these two sides that produces such horrifying behavior. So, if you try to intervene in the night terror by hugging the child without first making a connection to his consciousness, he may interpret the hugging as being chained or imprisoned, or being crushed by a devil or monster. If you try to speak or start yelling to get through to him, what he might see and hear will be like a scene from some horror movie that even adults could not bear to sit through.

Although we may never know what it is that the toddler actually experiences when these terrors occur, the gist of it is clear from what parents tell us. While still stuck within the night terror, the child seems to interpret the parents' gestures as threatening, if he acknowledges them at all.

Parents may wonder, "Why name the fear?" Although we cannot be certain exactly what effect *naming the fear* has on the child, judging by the testimonies of many parents, naming it seems to offer a life-line to the child. Perhaps verbalizing it opens a door between the unconscious and the conscious, and the child is able to walk out of hell. The naming somehow transforms his feeling (terror) into words. Just what is going on in the child's brain? I believe that the verbal reference triggers the cortex into overriding the hypothalamus. In other words, it triggers the rational brain into overriding the instinctual or emotional brain. There is ample evidence that it is possible for us to interpret words we hear when we are asleep, and there is support for this in parents' reports of their experiences. I myself find that I wake very easily at night if one of my children is making sounds that indicate any discomfort (whereas normally it would take trumpets next to my ears to get me out of bed). *For the Stramonium, what gets through is the word that names the fear, the exact trigger they can recognize. To open the door you need the one key that fits.*

Naming the fear can not only stop a particular night terror but also minimize future episodes. Since the unconscious wreaks havoc as it erupts through to the conscious level, each subsequent night terror enlarges the hole or breach that the unconscious rushes through. But as these attacks are reduced or prevented, the child can begin to feel increasingly safe. The safer he feels, the less fearful, the less violent, the less *Stramonium*, he becomes. It seems a reconciliation of the conscious with the unconscious has begun. There is a suturing of the breach between the two.

**How will the remedy affect the child with night terrors?** Potentially, in two ways. The first is the one we are looking for—the simple cure. "After the remedy Paul has been able to go to sleep by himself for the first time. He doesn't check for monsters anymore. He doesn't have to be with us at night so much. Nighttimes are better. He goes to sleep by himself and stays asleep. He seems more restful in his sleep now. He goes to sleep at night and naptime without my having to lie down with him." Months later, Joan reports that her son is still "falling asleep well and staying asleep, not waking in the middle of the night or grinding his teeth, not having the night terrors or other fears associated with sleep."

But there can also be an opposite response to the remedy. This is sometimes observed in very violent children who, previous to the remedy, did not have night terrors. However, after taking it, the child goes through a difficult period of both nightmares and night terrors. Alexis says of her daughter, "She would scream out loud and cry afterwards." These dreams usually start occurring in conjunction with the child becoming less violent. *As the external violent behavior decreases, the night terrors increase, acting as a pressure valve for the unconscious.* In these violent children, before the remedy, the *Stramonium* unconscious had full reign and so the child acted out his violence. But partway through the healing process, the conscious mind develops some impulse control, enabling the child to control his violence during the day. During sleep, however, the unconscious still wins out, for it is at this time that the child's newly gained control weakens, while the impulses remain strong. Thus a struggle now rages between the unconscious and the conscious, between the hypothalamus and the cortex, and between deep sleep and full awakening. As the healing progresses and the acting out lessens, the night terrors increase for a time, until eventually the child's impulses are not as strong. From this point on, these impulses can be sufficiently integrated by the child, who now begins to exhibit much calmer behavior, with neither violence during the day nor terrors at night.

*To summarize this portion, for me* **the night terrors really exemplify the Stramonium cycle.** *There is a time during sleep that the child partially wakes and becomes confused by this half-awake, half-asleep state (the confusion segment). The confusion leads to fears developing (the fear segment). To escape from the fear, he needs to move. This leads to all the striking behaviors as well as the urination (the violent overreaction segment) which leads to a desire to close down and not be touched (the closing off segment) because of gruesome images (the shut down/ dead segment).*

# STRAMONIUM

## General Sleep Symptoms

In addition to the pre-sleep fears and the night terrors, still other nighttime problems can occur. The child may exhibit a very **restless sleep** with **tossing, turning and waking up.** While most children's wakings are tumultuous, there are some children who wake up peacefully, ask for water, wait as if for dawn to arrive, and sleep again. I have discovered that *Stramonium* has **marked midnight** and **2 a.m. aggravations**. These are the two most likely times for the child to awaken or to experience night terrors.

Due to restlessness, no one consistent sleep position will be apparent. Quite a few of these children sleep on their back, or in the knee to chest position, or on their abdomen (as does *Medorrhinum*). However, you may find that, soon after the remedy is given, a child who had no preference will now desire to sleep on his abdomen. Further, like *Medorrhinum*, he may be so warm that he sleeps fitfully and uncovers his whole body.

The *Stramonium* child who is experiencing a great deal of emotional or neurological turmoil will grind his teeth during sleep, like *Tuberculinum*. This will be noticeable especially during an upper respiratory tract infection. If the child senses that he is being abandoned, he will often moan imploringly or whine "Mommy" in his sleep. Even though he is not having a nightmare, he may be fearing a loss of some kind.

As alluded to before, the *Stramonium* child may wet the bed until a very late age. This is a problem, not only because of the wetness triggering his fear of water and helping to induce a night terror, but also because of potential social criticism.

These children may also walk, cry, and talk in their sleep, independent of night terrors. They may do unusual things, such as have conversations in their sleep, or get up and urinate in the room. *Stramonium* has been known to take the bedsheets off or to crawl on the floor during sleep.

If the child feels unsafe, he may burrow himself into his blankets. This can cause profuse perspiration—mostly on the head and upper torso. **Perspiration during sleep is often observed in this remedy, especially on the head.**

The *Stramonium* child may exhibit some neurological symptoms during sleep. Most common are **twitching** and **jerking,** as well as **seizures.** These *neurologic Stramonium* children sleep in a slightly opisthotonic posture, with head drawn backward and off to one side.

# SLEEP

Unfortunately, if the child feels turmoil during the night, it is the parent who faces the turmoil in the morning. ***Stramonium* can be as irritable as *Tuberculinum*, *Medorrhinum*, or *Nux vomica* in the morning.** A mother enters her five year old's bedroom and says, "Good morning, Ernie." Ernie growls, "Don't talk to me! Get out of my room!" The mother becomes discouraged because she knows that for the next hour her son will scream, hit himself or others, or throw things, and in general be dissatisfied with everything. "Why does he put himself through this?" the parents ask the homeopath. "It doesn't seem like he is enjoying hurting us. Mostly, it seems like he's torturing himself." But it is no wonder that the child feels this way in the morning. As he begins to awaken he may still be experiencing aspects of his unconscious semi-sleep state. Thus he may still be somewhere between the conscious and the unconscious, trapped in that duality, just as he was in the night terror.

This chapter began by stating that the sleep of the child offers so many confirmatory symptoms that it would be unusual to find a *Stramonium* child not exhibiting some of these traits. **We have seen that the conscious and the unconscious, pulling against each other, can account for the fear, terror, and horrible dreams these children have at night, for it is at night that the balance between the conscious and the unconscious shifts. As the conscious side weakens and lets go, the unconscious side strengthens its grip and reigns. The conscious side becomes frantic as it loses control, and that is when the *Stramonium* symptoms come into full play.**

# *Body*

## HEAD

*Stramonium* is one of the main remedies to consider for children with **organic brain diseases, especially if they have developed any of the behaviors mentioned in the *Mind or Sleep* sections**. Children with **hydrocephalus, meningitis,** or **strokes,** with their respective after-effects, may need *Stramonium*. **Head injuries** are also a common etiology, though I have found that it is a **left-sided head injury** in particular that most commonly puts people into a *Stramonium* state. One confirmatory symptom to look for is that after the event there may have been a personality change in which aspects of any or all the major types of behaviors mentioned previously began to be evident. Mostly they will exhibit autistic traits, violent outbursts or issues dealing with evil.

Molly, who is fifteen years old, serves as an extreme example. When she was twelve, she was involved in an auto accident. The left side of her head crashed into the windshield, leaving her unconscious for a day. After that she developed seizures. While her parents are concerned about the seizures, what worries them most is the change in her behavior and personality ever since the accident. Her father continues: "She was an average kid, though maybe a little quiet. Now she is like no other kid I've ever met. In fact she's more like a vampire than anything else. She spends the evenings alone in her room and goes to sleep really late, then she stays asleep way into the morning. And she doesn't like the sun. In fact, three years ago she pulled the blinds on the window, and they've never been opened since. She no longer has friends; they all think she's weird. And she doesn't even care. She spends the day reading horror novels and writing little plays and stories that are really creepy. All the stories are about blood, carnage, entrapment, or defiling dead bodies. This is really sick stuff to be coming out of a fifteen year old who used to be an average kid. I know this all comes from the head injury and that I should think of it in the same way I do the seizures, but the way she behaves is really, really scary, really sick.

# STRAMONIUM

What will become of her three years from now, when she can legally be on her own? What kind of life will she choose?" Molly's history, though extreme, exemplifies the *Stramonium* response to a head injury: a change of personality, bringing forth either a demonic or a fearful side, along with the neurologic symptoms.

There are two other groups of symptoms that *Stramonium* covers regarding the head. One group deals with the nervous system, though most of these symptoms are included in the **Generalities** section at the end of the book. The other group of symptoms deals with headaches.

## Headaches

*Stramonium,* like *Belladonna,* affects the brain in such a way as to cause congestion which leads to headaches. Most of the time, the young child will not inform the parent that he is having a headache. It may therefore be very difficult to understand that he is behaving the way he is *because of the pain he is experiencing*. What *is* observed in the child, however, is a temper tantrum in which he screams and throws himself every which way. Occasionally, the child will try to relieve the discomfort by pressing his fingers into those parts of the head where the headaches most often occur—the temple, occiput, or forehead. These pains seem to be as severe as those in *Chamomilla, Lachesis, Tarentula hispanica,* or *Lyssinum,* driving the child to act irrationally. In some cases, the child will hit his head and neck, roll on the ground, and reach a point of irrational madness in which he bites himself and others. From the time they are around eight years old and onward, *Stramonium* children who have congestive headaches may say that they want to kill themselves because of the pain.

Children who have had meningitis, hydrocephalus, head injuries or a stroke experience the same type of headache, but may not be able to express themselves regarding this state. Again, the inconsolable shrieking, the head pounding, and the digging into a part of the skull with his hands, should signal to you the presence of a headache. Sometimes the parents, unaware of what the problem may be, try a headache medicine that stops the behavior, confirming all the more that the child feels head pain, as opposed to simply being unruly or out of control.

During the headache the head may become congested and hot. The extremities, hands and feet, on the other hand, may become cool. This can be extremely confusing since the *Belladonna* headache shares exactly the same description. A differentiating point is that the congestive headache (with uneven distribution of the blood and heat) is essential to *Belladonna*, whereas, if present in *Stramonium*, it will be less extreme. The opposite will be true in comparing the *behaviors* of *Stramonium* and *Belladonna*. Though the behaviors of the two may be similar, they will be more extreme in *Stramonium*.

The modalities of the headache will depend on the cause. In the congestive type of headache, warm applications and getting hot for any reason, such as being in a warm room, will aggravate the headache, while cold applications and fresh air will ameliorate it. But in the neuralgic type of headache, heat will help while cold will aggravate. Light aggravates all the headaches. In order to keep discomfort at a minimum, the child wants to be in a dark room and prefers not to have to move, since jarring motion also aggravates.

Accidentally hitting or bumping the head causes an interesting reaction in this remedy. While most children who accidentally hit their head will cry and fuss, it is very common for *Stramonium* to fall apart completely, to the point of an inconsolable temper tantrum. To an observer, the tantrum appears all too similar to the night terror behavior.

Although some *Stramonium* children are hypersensitive to pain, others seem to be oblivious to it. In fact, the parents of some *Stramonium* children report that they can get hit rather hard and still seem to not feel it. This illustrates the famous symptom, **painlessness of complaints that normally should hurt.**

**Thus *Stramonium* is notable for opposite reactions to pain—on the one hand being oversensitive to pain and on the other hand not feeling pain.** Both can be understood quite easily. In one situation, the injury triggers the type of unconscious response that has already been mentioned. In the other situation, the child is so self-absorbed that the injury does not register; it affects the body, but fails to penetrate through to the world in which the child's senses are operating at the time.

In a sense, the two behaviors mirror the familiar image of a conflict between two sides. On the one side is the child who is lost deep within the unconscious, as if in hell, as if dead. This side does not feel any pain.

STRAMONIUM

The other side is struggling to stay out of hell, trying to grasp for life, and is terribly frightened. This side feels pain far too intensely.

**Symptoms Within the Nervous System**

The symptoms within the nervous system mostly relate to what happens to the head during seizures. As mentioned at the beginning of the **Head** section, there are several causes that will traumatize the brain and many of these traumas cascade, to later cause seizures. If the child is old enough to express it or if the parents are observant, they may notice that the seizures begin with the child feeling a type of aura just before the attack. The child may touch or hit his head, claiming to feel 'funny' in his head.

During or after an actual trauma or inflammation, if the child is left with seizures, certain postures of the head are common. In one, the head is drawn or turned to one side or to the back (as in a localized motor area), or, if more severe, the whole back will be drawn backwards (as in opisthotonos).

**Jerking the head off the pillow** is a famous keynote of the remedy. If you see a child or adult that yanks his head up off the pillow during sleep, or during any form of semi-consciousness, strongly consider *Stramonium*. It should be noted, however, that this symptom is not as common, or as reliably present, as some of the materia medicas would suggest.

A behavior that is observed in *Helleborus* and *Tuberculinum* is also possible: the child may hit his head on the ground or roll his head into the pillow. This behavior, in meningitis, is so commonly ascribed to *Helleborus* that one may automatically think of only that remedy. However, the *Helleborus* child will often be unconscious and sleepy, whereas the *Stramonium* child will more likely be wild and fearful.

# VERTIGO

The several keynotes of *Stramonium* involving vertigo are not commonly seen in children, especially the symptom of vertigo if entering, standing in, or walking in the dark, However, a behavior which comes closest to that of vertigo may be observed in a child, usually two to five years of age, who appears to reel and swagger to and fro while acting silly, making jokes to

BODY

himself, seemingly unaware both of the homeopath and of the parent who is restraining the child in an effort to keep him from destroying the office.

# EYES

### Expression

The eyes of *Stramonium* provide several keynotes as well as common pathologies. Most particular are the various forms of expression that can be read in the stare of a *Stramonium* child. There is the **autistic stare,** in which the eyes either look away or look right through you with a fixedly wide, open stare, as if the child does not see you, or is in a world that you do not inhabit. In the **terror stare** the eyes are wide open with pupils fully dilated, as if the person has just seen his soul being ripped away from him. Lastly, the eyes may express a **look of evil.**

In the look of evil, the eyes take on a wild, shiny, almost gleaming quality. The pupils dilate and the whites glisten. There is a playful aspect to the stare, as of a madman who has cornered an innocent (in this case, the parents) and is toying with them, while in his mind he is leafing through a catalog of tortures to decide which he will inflict on his prey. It is the look of the possessed, of rage about to be unleashed. It is truly a look that sends shivers through anyone who has seen it. Seeing that stare one understands the parents' plight, who rightfully feel as if they are losing their baby to a monster.

I always look at the child very carefully, as I feel that his expression should in some way fit his real pathology. The expression itself shows the different aspects of *Stramonium*. The 'as if dead' aspect can be seen in the staring. The terror aspect fits the child who is in shock or disbelief of becoming possessed, whereas the look of evil fits someone who has already become possessed.

### Nervous System

Other symptoms observed in *Stramonium* have to do with nervous system disorders. If mild, there can be a nervous **twitch** around the eyelids; if more severe, there can be a great deal of **blinking.** Quite commonly, you

## STRAMONIUM

may find the child to be cross-eyed, most often with a convergent **strabismus.** These symptoms are even more useful indicators, and especially relevant if the child was a normal sighted child who, after experiencing a fright, then became cross-eyed or developed double vision or frequent blinking. Translated into the language of the cycle: a shock leads the child into the presentiment of death segment, which pushes him into the fear segment and needing to do something, but in so doing, there is an overshoot which causes the eyes to develop their nervous system symptoms. Strabismus that develops after a DPT vaccination is also likely to respond to *Stramonium*. A minority of these children may be either near or far-sighted from an early age.

As an aside, the *Stramonium* child who has eye symptoms in addition to behavioral and psychological difficulties, is a perfect candidate for Behavioral Optometry. These practitioners re-pattern the visual skills, helping the child to understand and incorporate what he sees. Such intervention can help, often miraculously, within a short period of time. Frequently, the hyper quality and the violence will stop shortly after this work begins.

Sometimes these disorders will be discovered in the patient's history. That is, eye problems may have been there since birth, along with other birth traumas, and after a great deal of therapy or surgery, may have disappeared or been greatly diminished. It is also possible that any of these nervous system disorders will crop up intermittently, appearing only during injury, fever, seizure, fright, or while stammering.

Another symptom that may be observed at times, is that the child will appear to lose control over the motion of his eyes. They seem to roll, moving in multiple directions. This happens especially when the child is giddy, out of control, or angry. Loss of eye control is also common during seizures and fevers.

Sometimes, instead of the eyes themselves moving from side to side, the eyelids will move, and in so doing, seem to make the eyes open or close of their own accord. During sleep or a night terror, and during a fever, the eyes will open. They will look as if they are staring at something inside the child's mind, something that cannot be articulated, except by an educated guess on your part. If you can figure out what that something is and name it, the eyes will begin to close again. It is as if just by naming it, that which is feared loosens its grip on the child. You can try naming different animals or anything of the color black. **The color black seems to produce such an intense impact on the child during the day, that he relives the *terror of* the black object, in some form, at night.**

At times, an opposite eye action will be observed, a closing of one or both eyes involuntarily. You may, for instance, have a three year old who, during the interview, will close one or both of his eyes. (I have noticed this happening most commonly in the left eye.) With the right eye open, he will turn his head to stare at you, or perhaps at the wall or ceiling, all the while giggling demonically.

## Light and Water

An important keynote of *Stramonium* is its relationship to light. Much literature focuses on the extreme **photophobia.** Truthfully, most of these children do not have an extreme form of it. However, in some circumstances, a child may complain of light hurting his eyes, often causing him to squint. This frequently happens in the car, when the reflection of sunlight on the glass irritates the *Stramonium's* eyes. The glare may even give an older child a headache. The younger child, confined in a car seat, may scream "Sssuuunnnn!" and cover his closed eyes, perhaps even distorting his face in an attempt to keep his eyes shut. Another time a child may be photophobic is during a fever, when his pupils are already dilated and he is slightly delirious. Lastly, during a bout of conjunctivitis, the eyes tend to be more photophobic.

A peculiar symptom, one that I have witnessed several times, is **temporary blindness.** It can be found in various situations, but the most common one is upon partial waking from sleep. The child may wake up screaming for his mother, "Mom! Help me! Come here! Turn on the lights!" (though the lights are on). The child screams that he cannot see and indeed may not see for up to a half hour. Another time blindness may be experienced is during high fevers. A child with a streptococcal infection may develop a headache, and aside from the headache, there is nothing particularly unusual about the infection until the child wakes screaming from a nap, terrified because he cannot see.

The fear of water, mentioned earlier in the *Mind: Fear* section, plays a role here. **The child has a great fear of water going in his eyes,** even during 'fun' times such as while in a pool or bathtub. If nothing else, the child fears the temporary blindness caused by the water. As mentioned before, it is interesting to me that, in relation to light, the child once again exhibits the two sides of the remedy. The unconscious side is 'half dead', sees nothing, shuns light, and is sensitive to light, while the conscious side is afraid of darkness and desires light, thus portraying this dual nature of *Stramonium* in the eyes.

## Infection

While it is not mentioned in any book, I have found that many *Stramonium* children will develop conjunctivitis. In fact, I have seen this so often that when I have to treat a child who has severe attention difficulties (with or without hyperactivity), along with frequent conjunctivitis, my mind quickly turns not only to *Medorrhinum*, but also to *Stramonium*. Because one usually does not think of *Stramonium* for this condition, the homeopath may mistakenly think the child has a true acute ailment and needs a separate remedy. The three most frequently mistaken remedies given in this situation are *Euphrasia*, *Pulsatilla*, and *Sulphur*. Of these, *Sulphur* is by far the most common mistake, since these two remedies may share many symptoms in such a child. Both remedy types may be extroverted. They may both think for themselves, be hot-blooded, be thirsty for cold, desire sweets, and have loose stools. If the children are old enough, both remedy types will describe a gritty, sandy sensation in the eyes. The eyes may become extremely red and itchy and begin to produce so much pus that in the mornings they are stuck together. The pus and tears make the area even redder. The eyes will also be aggravated in a warm room.

# EARS

## Infection and Pain

Recurrent ear infections are a common chief complaint of *Stramonium* patients. I mention this point because frequently it is tempting to give a different remedy at this time, a remedy that fits the ear itself and not the patient. *Stramonium* can be prescribed for an acute ear infection, for recurrent ear infections, or for the after-effects of an ear infection.

Though *Stramonium* appears rarely in the *Ear* section of the repertory,

I have used it frequently during acute earaches. The general state of the patient may resemble a combination of *Arsenicum album* and *Belladonna*, especially the latter. By looking carefully, one will find many symptoms similar to *Belladonna*. The sudden onset, waking up screaming, high fever, red face, a sensitivity to noise, throbbing ear pains, and, if severe enough, a consciousness level approaching that of delirium. The fact that many times the ear and the tympanic membrane are red only adds to the confusion. While this latter symptom may be a keynote of several remedies, *Stramonium* is not even listed in the rubrics: **EAR: Discoloration, redness; EAR: Inflammation, inside;** and **EAR: Inflammation, media,** though it should be. I have added it in my repertory.

Fortunately, there are three major distinctions that should help to differentiate *Stramonium* from *Belladonna*. First, if the ear pain is neuralgic and is ameliorated by heat and bundling up, it will fit *Stramonium*, but if it is congestive and tends to be aggravated by heat, it will fit both *Belladonna* and *Stramonium*.

Secondly, and of greater significance, there is much more fear, restlessness, and nighttime aggravation in *Stramonium*. In this respect, it resembles *Arsenicum album*. While *Belladonna* may have fears during fever, *Stramonium's* fears are much more intense, bordering on terror. The fear will often not be expressed verbally, but it can be observed in the terrified look on the child's face. He may also become extremely clingy, wanting to hold on to the parent, or even desire to be carried. At the same time, however, he may be averse to being kissed or caressed, and may actually be mean or occasionally violent toward the parents. So once again we see the two sides of *Stramonium*, even in the ear pain: the fearful side, clinging and not wanting to be alone and the half demonic side wanting to torture and enjoying aloneness. When I speak of children in pain, I would definitely add *Stramonium* to the rubrics: **MIND: Company, aversion, dreads being alone, yet; MIND: Company, desire for, yet treats them outrageously.**

Lastly, *Belladonna*, during the ear infection with fever, has as a keynote symptom a hot head with cold extremities. *Stramonium* may have the hot head but the extremities may not be as cold as in *Belladonna*. As long as the prescriber checks the relative temperature of the face and extremities, the confusion as to which remedy should be given will be lessened.

# STRAMONIUM

A perfect example of a *Stramonium* earache is the one that two year old Sally had. It began with Sally waking up at 2 a.m., vomiting and coughing, screaming that her left ear hurt. Each time she coughed it would make her vomit again. She was clearly frightened; her expression was one of fear, with wide open eyes. She was clinging to her father. She was capricious, crying that she wanted this and then that, though nothing satisfied her. She was bossy with both her mother and father. First she wanted one parent and then she wanted the other, demanding that the first should leave the room. She would sit staring at the wall like a zombie, and then shift into a state of high energy, going from one place to another. She would not go back to sleep (and in fact did not nap during the day any more). The only recent occurrence that the parents noted as unusual was that, the day before, an adult wearing a mask had scared her. In this case, we find **the following points to confirm *Stramonium*: the screaming, fear, fright, and clinging that fit the one side of *Stramonium* and the demanding, nastiness of the other side of the remedy.** This capricious behavior is caused by the two equally strong sides vying for prominence.

The fear on the *Stramonium* child's face may be caused by two things. First, the pain may be so torturous that he might not understand that it is caused by an ear infection and thus not be able to endure it. But even if he is old enough to be able to pinpoint the cause, the severity of the pain itself may open up his unconscious. He may experience the fear as if he were a prisoner being tortured in some God-forsaken jail. He may even writhe on the floor, trying to escape the intense pain in his head, but to no avail. A child may actually have a seizure during an ear inflammation. The parents and doctors are seldom sure whether the seizure is due to the fever or to the extreme amount of pain that the child seems to be going through. Sometimes when they have to perform a spinal tap to rule out a meningitis, it sends the child still further into a *Stramonium* state. From that day on, even after the earache and fever are gone, the child no longer acts the same; he becomes less confident, more fearful and less communicative.

The second reason for the fearful look is that the fever may be affecting some portion of the limbic system in his brain and he could enter a hallucinatory delirium. In this state he sees "scary, hairy, ghostly" things that make his mere survival seem questionable.

I wonder if we, doctor and parent, could just put ourselves in the child's position for one moment. Can we really expect a two year old with a fever to be able to differentiate between whether he has a severe ear pain or whether he is being ritually abused and beaten in the ear/head? The fears, insecurity, or violence that can develop out of the experience of feeling as if tortured (by this pain) can, in itself, be enough of a reason for needing *Stramonium*, as this scenario creates the feeling or fear of being injured. See rubrics: **MIND: Fear, injured, of being;** and **MIND: Delusion, injury, is about to receive.**

While many attribute the cause of ear infections to eating too many sweets, sleeping with the bottle, or drinking too much juice, I would also argue that some ear infections commonly begin after a *Stramonium's* parent goes back to work. Perhaps this leaves the child feeling abandoned, a significant point of stress for *Stramonium*.

One of the reasons *Stramonium* is listed in the rubric: **GENERALITIES: Side, crosswise, left upper and right lower** is that *Stramonium* is listed as stronger for the left ear and nose and for the right chest and bronchi. In differentiating *Stramonium* from *Belladonna*, it may help to note that, while earaches may occur for both in either ear, *Belladonna* is typically prone to right-sided earaches, while *Stramonium* is more apt to have them on the left side.

### Hearing

The parents of the 'autistic trait' type may tell you that their child seems not to be in communication with others. Parents have to repeat their questions, commands, or requests several times before the child responds, if he responds at all. The parents may also have taken the child for auditory testing, attributing the difficulty to impaired hearing due to fluid in the ear, to a serous otitis media, or to poor auditory integration within the brain.

# NOSE

*Stramonium* does not seem to affect the nose in any unusual ways. Some children do not have any nose complaints, while others develop recurrent colds that cease after the remedy is given. If present, these colds are often nondescript. They may even seem trivial compared to the other worries which the parents have. They may complain that the child often has a runny nose. Commonly, the runny nose dries up, thereby obstructing the child's breathing. Such discomfort occurs most especially at night. It may discharge in the cold air and when eating. During the initial heat phase of a severe bronchitis or pneumonia, the nose, throat, and bronchi feel very dry. The nose may be so dry that the child develops nosebleeds, especially at night.

# MOUTH

### Stammering

One of the most striking aspects of *Stramonium* is seen in the speech. *Stramonium* is well known in the treatment of adults and children who stammer. Above all other remedies, *Stramonium* allows observation, almost palpable, of the connection between the tongue, the mouth, and the speech centers of the brain. To witness a *Stramonium* stammer is often so startling to the observer that he may fear the person is having a seizure.

Usually, the stammering is not present when speech is first developing in the child. The stuttering may frequently be attributed to a fright and its aftermath. A parent reporting this symptom said, "My child has been stuttering for the past four months, ever since he saw a witch in a haunted house. In general, he stammers most predictably whenever he is afraid or reprimanded or excited. He begins speaking but then gets stuck in the middle of his sentence. Whenever he stutters, his eyes are wide open, and he blinks a lot." Some children become so excited while speaking that they will speak faster and faster, and suck up air as they talk.

### Teeth

Dentition is a common time to find the *Stramonium* child's symptoms aggravated. His behavior while teething may be his very worst. He may scream inconsolably for hours at a time, become violent, scratch his mother's face and breast, have an increase in seizure activity, or grind his teeth. He may also develop diarrhea or a respiratory tract infection. As can be seen from the above symptoms, *Stramonium* at this time will act in a manner similar to *Tuberculinum* and may be mistaken for it, as well as for *Cina* and *Chamomilla*.

Another chronic symptom shared with *Tuberculinum* is the teeth grinding that appears in sleep, especially during upper respiratory tract infections. And the chronic symptoms of a dry mouth leading to high thirst reminds one of *Sulphur, but as long as the homeopath focuses on the reason behind the disturbance of the child, for instance, seeing that it is the overreactive nervous segment that is behind the stammering or the stress of teething, he will arrive at Stramonium as the remedy.* However, if he focuses only on local particular symptoms or even only on physical general symptoms, then mistakes in prescribing such remedies as *Tuberculinum, Cina, Chamomilla,* and *Sulphur* will occur.

**Canker Sores**

Some of these children have a tendency towards canker sores in the mouth. It is a small point, but it can throw the case awry, because this tendency may cause a strong aversion to acidic foods such as tomatoes and citrus, which, in turn, can be mistakenly analyzed as a strong aversion to sour. In reality, if such an aversion exists in a *Stramonium* child, I would suspect that the digestive tract is sensitive to acids. This would point to a local aggravation, as opposed to a physical general condition, which usually is weighted more heavily in the analysis of the patient.

# FACE

**Color**

As with the eyes, we may observe a great deal of what the child is going through right there in his face. In terms of color, the face is often either very pale or very red, once again mirroring the two sides of the remedy. On the one side is paleness, the part is going toward death, while on the other side is redness, the part so full of life. The pale face often comes after an upper respiratory tract infection. One parent's description: "My child had a healthy glow to his skin until he got mumps. Since then he is positively ashen." This also can apply to whooping cough.

The reddish color often accompanies the child's emotional turmoil, fevers, or seizures, comparable to *Belladonna*. A slight differential is that often, during an upper respiratory tract infection, the face of *Belladonna* will be plethoric, the redness being caused by the fullness of blood, while the *Stramonium* face will manifest the kind of redness caused by the chafing of skin that at times accompanies such infections. This chafed red color may also be found in allergic children, mostly on the cheeks, and is aggravated by eating the offending foods, usually dairy, citrus, or wheat.

**Infection**

*Stramonium* may also be thought of during mumps. A *Stramonium* child's behavior may worsen after a bout of the mumps or after an MMR vaccination. Also possible are facial skin infections, which are red in color and lead to erysipelas and delirium.

**Nervous System**

Nervous tics and twitches may be seen in the face. Sometimes, as in *Staphysagria*, these will occur when the child is staring out into space, but more often they will accompany or follow a fearful state, such as when a father is yelling at the child or when the child is afraid of water getting on his face, or afraid of being near the ocean. At such fearful times the expression on the face will be that of a caged and terrified wild animal. However, when the child loses control and becomes violent, the look will change to that of a fierce beast coming in for the kill. With his mouth wide open he grimaces and laughs, seemingly staring into the great beyond.

One symptom mentioned as common in past materia medicas is that the *Stramonium* face bears a wrinkled forehead. In practice, we do not find it as commonly as one would have thought. It is most often observed in a neurologic condition (as in a seizure state or if unconscious) or sometimes when the child, feeling challenged by the homeopath's interview, becomes fearful or nervous because he fails to understand the questions. This can lead to confusion with the remedy *Lycopodium*. In *Lycopodium*, the overall impression during this wrinkling is one of anxiety, whereas in *Stramonium* you may sense curiosity, fear, and a certain tension. You might even feel as if the child will pounce on you unless you diffuse the tension.

BODY

# THROAT

*Stramonium* sore throats and cases of **tonsillitis** begin, for the most part, with a throat that feels rough and is very dry. The voice may become hoarse, after which a cold develops, perhaps changing into a more severe ailment such as tonsillitis, with swollen cervical glands, or **even bronchitis**. The tonsillitis may be accompanied by a high fever, sharp pains, and a reddish-colored throat that resembles *Belladonna*. The swelling of the tonsils and glands can make it too painful to swallow. The infection may also be accompanied by delirium or seizures and may make sleep problematic. The child may wake from bed-wetting, from bad dreams (of wolves for example), or with an accentuated fear of the dark. *Pulsatilla* and *Sulphur* may mistakenly be given at this time. Even though quite ill, he may still become whiny, or clingy. He may ask the parent pleadingly, "Do you love me?" (making the homeopath think, "Perhaps the child needs *Pulsatilla*?") But then he decides to hit the parent and *Pulsatilla* is discarded. Another possibility is that the child may suddenly become warm, red-lipped, and thirsty for very cold water (all common symptoms of *Sulphur*). After considering giving *Sulphur*, you notice that the child has developed a new habit, holding his penis incessantly. Since this is a common symptom for *Stramonium, Sulphur* can be discarded.

*Stramonium* is listed very strongly for many types of paralysis of the throat, as well as for spasms, constrictions, and choking. These are rarely seen in the pediatric population, and if found should make one think of other remedies first, such as *Hyoscyamus* and *Lachesis*. There is, however, one common scenario that would make one think of *Stramonium*, that of a child who has difficulty swallowing and consequently develops fears and behavior problems. An example of this could be a child who is fine until he receives a DPT vaccination. Soon after, he develops swallowing difficulties, perhaps even choking, and then becomes fearful and begins to act out violently.

Alan's story is slightly different. His throat began to close up after taking an antibiotic for impetigo, which resulted in an anaphylactic reaction. He was rushed to an emergency room where he was given medicine to stop the reaction. I believe that he entered into a *Stramonium* layer from that unfortunate and frightful experience. Subsequently, Alan became reclusive, did not want to play with other children, was fearful at night, and developed frequent attacks of rage.

Ulcers in the throat, so painful that the infant can not nurse, cry out, or swallow properly, may likewise lead the child into a *Stramonium* state. This can be attributed to the shock of the pain and perhaps as well to the inability to express his anguish.

### Voice

Many *Stramonium* children develop recurring respiratory tract infections. The voice is often affected, becoming hoarse and possibly staying so throughout the entire winter. When I have asked the parents about this hoarseness, I have been surprised that they often do not even notice the quality of the voice. Upon reflection, they frequently ascribe the hoarseness to the child's constant screaming and yelling, and suggest that perhaps he is developing laryngitis simply from yelling too much.

## LOWER RESPIRATORY TRACT

### Bronchitis

Most *Stramonium* children will have a **history of repeated coughs and bronchitis** treated many times with antibiotics. One observation that I have made, after treating so many emotionally challenging children, is that many of them develop a certain cough. This applies not only to *Stramonium* but also to most other remedies for truly violent or hyperactive children. What is remarkable about this is that most of the coughs bear a striking resemblance to a lingering pertussis cough. Since the symptoms of this particular cough are so similar to those of pertussis, and further, since I have seen so many children need *Stramonium* either after receiving the vaccine or after catching whooping cough, I have begun to consider, of late, that there exists a relationship between the pertussis vaccine and *Stramonium*. Interestingly, whooping cough is called the 'black cough' in various countries around the world.

The chief complaint of a child who needs *Stramonium* may very likely be a cough. **This cough will be dry, spasmodic, and teasing.** The child seems not to be aware of it and continues to act his usual self. The parents worry, however, because the cough seems to them to be relentless. They go to their orthodox physician, who tells them that the child has a viral infection and needs to take an antibiotic just in case a bacterial superinfection occurs. Unfortunately, either the antibiotic fails to achieve the anticipated results or else its apparent gains seem to disappear once it is no longer being administered. The parents then wonder if the interminable coughing may be due to a food allergy or perhaps an airborne allergy. I have seen all these reasons attributed to the same basic cough. Even during sleep this incessant cough may continue.

Many *Stramonium* boys, in some cases beginning as young as infancy, seem to develop frequent **bronchitis** as well. Often there will be a history of an initial croup or pertussis, in which case the child may either have kept the barking cough or may experience its recurrence after eating too many sweets, being frightened, or becoming slightly chilled in a swimming pool. Again, some of the symptoms may resemble *Belladonna*, though they may also resemble *Spongia tosta, Drosera,* or *Nux vomica*. At first this barking cough may sound dry and croupy and may actually make the child retch. The adolescent may complain that his whole chest feels extremely dry inside and that breathing is painful. There are accompanying signs and symptoms such as a high fever, but again, what the parents worry about, and most complain of, is the intense and persistent cough which seems to be ever present.

The cough may be aggravated by lying down, during sleep, and from being in the cold air. It grows worse in the evening, especially at night, and worse also when the child wakes up in the morning. It may already have been treated several times with different acute remedies, such as *Bryonia alba* or *Drosera*. These remedies may slightly alter the cough in character or modality, but it persists nonetheless. Over time, during the intense part of the fever, the child will start to drool and sweat at night, which will prompt one to think of *Mercurius solubilis*. All these acute remedies are incorrect, the constitutional remedy being the only one called for.

As the cough lingers, it gradually changes from dry and croupy to more phlegmy, sometimes producing a loose yellow expectoration and then becoming dry again. This situation may last for months. Many parents complain that their child has had a cough the whole winter long. I have noticed that while *Pulsatilla* or *Sulphur* are often prescribed at this point, both remedies seem to merely palliate the cough, only to have it return. Or, just as likely, the remedy will change some of the modalities, while the cough itself lingers on.

Another remedy that can be mistaken for *Stramonium* in the respiratory symptoms is *Phosphorus*. During bronchitis and pneumonia, these two remedies share the symptom of oppression on the chest. They both may say, "It feels as if someone is pressing on my chest," or, "it feels like I have a weight on my chest."

Often, after experiencing one acute chest bronchitis or tracheitis, the child will seem different. He may develop fears, or be unable to concentrate, and may have a shorter attention span. He may also lose appetite and weight. Although he may be taking many antibiotics, none of them seem to stop this merry-go-round of infection, antibiotic, infection, antibiotic—a cycle which has been in effect ever since he had whooping cough or shortly after he was given the pertussis vaccine.

One such child, Valerie, came to see me when she was seven years old, with the chief complaint of night terrors which began when she was three. Shortly after a vaccination, the child developed an upper respiratory tract infection. It began with hoarseness, but quickly settled into her chest with a bronchitis, rattling cough, high fever, and listlessness. The bronchitis finally resolved but she was left with a post-nasal catarrh. Soon after that she began to grind her teeth and experience night terrors. One dose of *Stramonium* 200C and she was back to her old self within two months.

## Pneumonia

Pneumonia may also be treated successfully with this remedy. While the repertory lists *Stramonium* for only the right side, either side is possible. Following a typical pneumonia, the child develops a high fever of approximately 104° which is accompanied at first by a cold, cough, or streptococcal throat infection. Shortly thereafter, the breathing becomes short, fast, and laborious.

In its early phase the cough is dry, like the spasmodic, teasing cough of bronchitis, but in pneumonia it may also cause a terrible headache and chest pain. It feels as if the ribs are bruised, or that they are separating from the sternum. Some patients may say that they feel as if someone is sitting on their sternum, or complain of a choking sensation and an oppression, which may be worse in the dark. They may become constipated during this dry phase. Thus far the remedy may sound like *Bryonia alba*, but the thirst will aid in the differentiation. While both remedies will crave ice cold drinks during this infection, *Stramonium* will cough more from the drink.

Another differentiating point is that *Bryonia alba* may enter into a delirium in which they wish to go home (even if they are at home), whereas characteristically in delirium, *Stramonium* will experience an accentuated fear of the dark, and become clingy and scared, because they see faces and devils and black animals. They may awaken in a state of fright, unable to describe the horror they have experienced. During the delirium, they may feel such terror that they want to get out of bed to escape their surroundings. Whenever you stop holding them, they begin to rise, trying to get away, and you then find yourself restraining them just as you might if they were having a violent temper tantrum or a dangerous night terror. As the infection develops, they begin to have more and more night sweats and a thick, white expectoration that eventually turns yellowy-green with bloody tinges.

## Asthma

Although not the most common chief complaint, asthma may nevertheless be present. The asthma consists of a spasmodic cough, and is associated with constriction of the chest. The shortness of breath worsens at night, while lying down, and from cold air and drink, as well as from frights and from animal dander or fur (from cats, for example). Older children may describe the sensation either as an oppression of the chest or as a difficulty in exhaling.

George's story is typical. George is three years old and has asthma. His respiratory difficulties began during a period of recurring croup. One time, during the croup, he was given antibiotics, and soon after began to wheeze and cough and had to be taken to the emergency room. Ever since that time, he has been caught in a cycle that lasts three to six weeks. The cycle is as follows. He develops a cold with a runny nose. Soon after that he begins to wheeze and have a dry tight cough that causes him to vomit. He wakes up with this asthma, becoming fearful and irritable, as well as fastidious. He is very contrary and begins hitting, biting, throwing objects and being mean to the animals. He loses his attention span, regresses to acting like a baby, and though becoming neat, yet is averse to bathing. Now his sleep is disturbed as well; he talks in his sleep, becomes restless, and wakes up because of bad dreams. Even though there are aspects of other remedies seen in cases like George's, remedies that are more well known for asthma, if you look at the overall case, you find many convincing symptoms for the *Stramonium* picture.

# STRAMONIUM

Some *Stramonium* children have a severe form of asthma as a chief complaint. Many of those children will have a history that may suggest that the child originally needed *Tuberculinum* or *Lycopodium* but with the first severe attack, the asphyxiation created such fear that he entered the *Stramonium* state and stayed there. When the child coughs, he says it feels as if he has a weight on his chest, or as if he is suffocating, which I equate with the side of *Stramonium* that is 'in the coffin'. For this type, the asthma becomes aggravated by anything that accentuates the buried, dead side of the battle, such as the dark, night, or sleep.

## Management of Asthma

I believe that when homeopaths look back over their *Stramonium* cases, they will find several occasions when, soon after the remedy was given, the patient developed a bronchitis while appearing to improve in general. After the bronchitis was treated with whatever remedy or remedies seemed appropriate, the case relapsed and the patient again needed *Stramonium*. I think that this **relapse occurs and the case goes awry because of the introduction of an unnecessary second remedy; a repeat of *Stramonium* would have sufficed in many of these cases.** But unfortunately *Stramonium* is not yet well known for such respiratory tract infections. In my practice, I have found that if a remedy *is* needed, repeating their constitutional remedy, *Stramonium*, at that time allows the patient to overcome the infection completely, as long as the general picture is unchanged, and if the patient *does* need a repetition and is not going to recover by himself.

Before leaving this discussion, I would like to suggest that, in many instances, respiratory tract infections play an important role in the body's attempt to stay healthy. **These multiple infections often serve as a pressure valve through which the body tries to redress an internal imbalance.** If allowed to do so, the balance of the child will be restored. This may explain why so many parents say that their otherwise obnoxious, violent, unrelenting child is an angel during these infections. Many such infections will develop after a shock to the child, often some event in which he feels abandoned, such as a parent leaving the house for a business trip, or the parents getting divorced. This throws him off balance. In treating these illnesses, the allopathic physician's method is an attempt to stop this venting, which in fact is the body's way of correcting an imbalance. But after such antipathic treatment, you may notice over time that the child is developing more and more symptoms on the mental/emotional plane. As homeopaths, we have all too often observed this unfortunate trend.

Moreover, once a correct homeopathic remedy is given, it is likely that as the mental/emotional realms begin to heal, the child will develop some infection—an earache, a cough, or perhaps bronchitis. If what we surmise is true, then the infection should not, in most circumstances, be treated with another remedy. While we absolutely wish to keep the child safe, I have observed **many wonderful beginnings lose their promise when the homeopath, trying to stop physical discomfort, gives a homeopathic remedy that only partially fits.** Occasionally, simply repeating the same remedy can be very effective. The best course of treatment is not to give a remedy, but instead to administer some natural treatment that will supply the body nourishment with which to heal, without interfering with the healing process.

Be forewarned. Sometimes the treatment of asthma with homeopathic medicine can be simple and so strikingly effective as to make one want to practice twenty-four hours a day, seven days a week to help everyone. **However, asthma is a potentially life-threatening disease, and many difficulties can arise, especially if the child has a complicated form of the disease. The treatment is best left to professional homeopaths who have experience with drug/drug interactions as well as with the long term management needed to eventually turn the medicated asthmatic child to the unmedicated no-longer asthmatic child.**

# STOMACH

### Appetite

Even the appetite can show the two sides of *Stramonium:* an increased appetite for the side that wants to live and a decreased appetite for the side that's trance-like. But most *Stramonium* appetites will decrease over time. One notable exception is if a child was starved earlier in life. In such an instance, he will have a voracious appetite. The reasons for the otherwise decreasing appetite may be several. A child may have attention difficulties or be too restless to sit at a table long enough to eat, and so stands and picks at his food. One parent reports, "He was a good eater but, ever since the DPT vaccination, I think he may be hypoglycemic because his actions are so violent and irrational. He has become so restless and such a picky eater, though. It's no wonder he doesn't eat." In these children, breakfast is the first meal to disappear. They are capricious, saying that they do not know what they want to eat. The older ones may tell you that they are nauseous in the morning and that looking at or even thinking about food may cause them to retch. One of the wonderful results of taking the remedy will be that the child gets back his previous good appetite.

### The Duality in Food Desires and Aversions

If the child has one particular food desire, it is sweets. **Most *Stramonium* children will have a very strong craving for sweets.** It will be underlined strongly in your case-taking. In fact, I have added it in bold type in my repertory. Sweets may aggravate the child's misbehavior and may cause loose stools. Other strong food cravings, though less common, may be for all types of dairy: cheese, ice cream, yogurt, and milk (especially cold). A subset of the infants will have projectile vomiting of milk and may be averse to or aggravated by breastfeeding. **There may be a strong craving for fruits, especially citrus, lemons and oranges.** A smaller group will crave raw vegetables or salt. However, some may be averse to vegetables, mostly to tomatoes or tomato sauce. Some crave fatty, smoked meats or salamis, while others are averse to tough meats and occasionally to eggs. More characteristic of *Stramonium*, especially of the ritualistic subtype, is a strong aversion to mixed-up foods, as is also to be observed, each for their own reasons, in *Natrum muriaticum, Calcarea carbonica,* and *Tuberculinum.*

Even though the materia medicas and repertories show *Stramonium* as being both thirsty and thirstless, **I have found that the vast majority of the children have a great thirst, especially for very cold water or even ice, and like juices such as orange or apple juice.** Differentiation should be made with *Sulphur, Medorrhinum* and *Veratrum album,* all of which crave ice and juice. And if you see a small appetite combined with a desire to drink, it will make the choice between *Stramonium* and *Sulphur* still more difficult since both remedies share these characteristics. In addition, the rubric: **STOMACH: Appetite, wanting, with thirst,** which is a keynote for *Sulphur*, is shared by *Stramonium* and should be added to it in italics. Also, *Stramonium* has in common with *Sulphur* and *Medorrhinum* a desire for alcohol, especially for beer; this can be seen in *Stramonium* children as young as three or four years old.

To conclude this section on food desires, aversions and thirst, there are two important points that will, I believe, help to clarify why *Stramonium* children have these particular food cravings. The first is that many of these patients have a strong miasmatic tendency and so share a great many symptoms with nosodes, or with the central remedies within those miasms. In fact, I find it is easy to classify *Stramonium's* cravings as a mixture, or combination, of those observed in *Medorrhinum,* in *Tuberculinum* and in the great antipsoric, *Sulphur.*

The second point has to do with the contradiction between cravings and aversions listed above. Many *Stramonium* individuals crave a particular food while others are averse to that same food. I pondered this fact for several years until I hit on the observation that those children who desire light and consolation and fear of the dark and of being alone, seemed to like the comfort foods, such as sweets and dairy, while those who were more violent and demonic craved lemons and were averse to or aggravated by comfort foods such as milk. This unusual observation, along with many others, will be explored in greater detail in my upcoming book on the homeopathic treatment of attention difficulties in children. For now, my purpose in listing the food cravings is not only to share unknown symptoms but also to again illustrate the two diametrically opposed sides of this remedy. Not only are their personalities opposites, but even their food cravings show this split.

## ABDOMEN

Abdominal complaints are mostly limited to stomach-aches that are either the chief complaint or just a symptom accompanying some other illness. There is nothing particularly distinctive about them and the remedy will rarely be confirmed in this area. However, I have noted several common

## STRAMONIUM

scenarios for *Stramonium* with regard to the abdomen. First, there is the abdominal complaint of a somatized fear which arises in anxious situations. For example, in children with night terrors, there can be stomach/abdominal pains before bedtime. Such pains will cease when the fears diminish. Secondly, there can be abdominal pain that precedes a bowel movement, a symptom shared with *Medorrhinum*. Abdominal pains may also accompany loose stools or diarrhea—the more severe the diarrhea, the more severe the pains. Lastly, there are abdominal pains that are probably more muscular in origin. I make this assumption both because heat ameliorates the pains and because they occur concomitantly with back pains.

## RECTUM

Most of the boys that need *Stramonium* will have a tendency toward loose stools. This makes the possibility of confusing *Stramonium* with *Tuberculinum* or *Sulphur* quite high, especially if you find it in a hyperactive, warm-blooded child who cannot sit still and who acts out. The loose stools may become frank diarrhea, in which the child dehydrates and becomes very ill. The diarrhea can be sour and offensive and cause the area around the anus to become sore and red. These last symptoms, along with the child's high thirst and warmth, further remind us of *Sulphur*.

The soft, loose and unpredictable nature of the toddler's stools may make toilet training very difficult. The stool may cause some emotional distress in the child. He hates to have his diaper changed, resisting and fighting with whoever is trying to change him. He fights against this, even though the loose stool is seeping out of the diaper onto his clothes or down his legs. Some of these children experience great difficulties in toilet training before receiving the remedy. But after *Stramonium* the stools become solid again and we come to see a proud child, happily involving himself in the training. Within a mere month, the toilet training can change from being a fierce struggle between the parent and child to a situation in which the child actually leads the effort.

Those children that are overly controlled, anxious, introverted, and compulsive, may desire to wipe carefully after a bowel movement, trying to keep the parts extremely clean. They may feel compelled to wash the anus and hands after every bowel movement.

Involuntary stools are possible if the child is delirious. In the repertory, *Hyoscyamus* is listed stronger for this symptom, but in clinical practice we more often see *Hyoscyamus* passing the stool for shock value or because of inattention due to excitement. In *Stramonium*, however, it occurs due to a physical condition, perhaps inflammation or fever, that affects the brain. It is not performed for its shock value but rather because the child is not himself aware of the stool.

If, for any reason, the child has a very high fever which affects the brain, he may dehydrate and become constipated as well as not pass urine, reminding us of *Apis mellifica*. The differentiating point is that during these states most often the *Stramonium* child will still be extremely thirsty for ice cold drinks, whereas the *Apis mellifica* child will be thirstless. The only exceptions occur in fevers that accompany upper respiratory tract infections, during which time the Tubercular side of *Stramonium* may cause the child to have loose stools, as described in the **Lower Respiratory Tract** section.

# URINARY SYSTEM

During fevers, it is common to see the urine output change. Some of the children will have an increased flow of urine. Others will have a decreased flow all the way to anuria, complete urinary suppression. You will most often witness, concurrent with anuria, a delirious state in which the child becomes violent or frightened.

As alluded to in the **Sleep** section, characteristic for some *Stramonium* toddlers is profuse urination at night. It may be too much for the diapers to hold, and as they begin to leak all over the bedclothes and mattress, the child will moan and may experience a night terror. A differentiating point is that often this profuse night urine is light-colored and odorless, as opposed to that of other remedies, which may have an offensive odor or stain the bedding.

STRAMONIUM

# BOYS

The boys often hold their genitals, either outright or by keeping a hand in the pocket. While some other remedies (especially *Hyoscyamus*) have this symptom more commonly, *Stramonium* can include this behavior. *Hyoscyamus* does this for two reasons—first and foremost as exhibitionism, to tease, and only secondarily as a nervous system response to stress. In contrast, *Stramonium* displays such behavior mostly as a nervous system response. It seems as though his hand is always on his penis, especially in violent young boys with attention and impulse control difficulties. The young child (even the toddler) may obsess over mom's and other women's breasts, reaching out and touching them. This may be observed in a weaned two year old. Even at seven or eight years of age, the child may use sexual language and obsess on sexual matters.

One of the difficulties that either begins or exacerbates the state of *Stramonium* may be from touching the genitals too forcefully. One example is eight year old Jonathan who after rubbing his uncircumcised penis too forcefully developed phimosis and balanitis, an infection of the foreskin that later extended to his whole penis. He was given antibiotics, to which he was allergic. His throat swelled and he was rushed to the hospital just as his breathing became compromised. Ever since that incident, Jonathan has been extremely fearful at night, and has taken to reading scary stories and dressing as a superhero. From several similar cases, in which *Stramonium* has cured the infection, I think that *Stramonium* should be added to the infection of the penis rubrics, such as **MALE: Inflammation; MALE: Inflammation, penis; MALE: Inflammation, penis, glans; MALE: Phimosis; MALE: Redness, glans;** and **MALE: Swelling, penis.**

The *Stramonium* boy may wish to never wear clothes at home and yet may be shy and proper in company. This can be observed in a seven year old showing sexual curiosity, wanting to know about sex and asking about it. This is the opposite of *Hyoscyamus* who will do or say anything just for its shock value. Needless to say, these *Stramonium* children wind up having sex at a young age.

A further symptom relating to the boy's anatomy may be a history of undescended testicles, where all sorts of treatments have been tried to encourage them to descend but each approach has failed, short of surgery.

Sometimes even homeopathy has failed after trying with remedies such as *Lycopodium* and *Baryta carbonica*. It is only following the surgery that the fears and behavior difficulties arise. Until that point no remedy can be found, simply because the *Stramonium* picture remains hidden and incomplete. It only emerges clearly after the surgery. In such a situation, if you have already tried several remedies, look carefully to see if indeed there were any keynotes for *Stramonium* (even if it seems unlikely) before the surgery, because much of the remedy picture may be missing in the earlier stages.

# GIRLS

A common complaint, though without a distinct keynote, has to do with the menses, which can be extremely painful for some girls, with the pain sometimes extending into the groin and thighs. If menses occurs during fever, the flow may stop and start, becoming offensive and dark. There may be pre-menstrual symptoms where the girl will become reclusive, cut herself with razors or knives, and exhibit violent or sexual behavior.

Sexual abuse may sometimes be found in the history of these girls. While this issue comes up more in treating adults, it also surfaces in teenage girls. Any of the following effects might be noted after such abuse. If the girl experienced fright along with the sexual abuse, she may begin to have terrible dreams about invasion of her body, of monsters ravaging her, or of being pursued by evil—any one of which may lead to a fear of going to bed at night. Another effect of abuse can be seen in the young girl who, due to the shock, has repressed all memories of it. It is possible that sexual abuse will shift her into a *Stramonium* layer, and even though she may not receive treatment at that time, she may, after a while, move into a different remedy layer. If she is then treated with the remedy for this newer layer, the *Stramonium* layer will suddenly be freed to surface, with all of its panic and bad dreams.

For such a girl, this is a layer that was repressed and has only now become available to be addressed. It is not surprising then, that she will say that only since taking the *Stramonium*, the second prescription, does she feel that her life is finally changing for the better. It seems to have meant little to her that with the previous remedy her asthma, migraines, or whatever complaint disappeared. The way I think of this situation is that the *Stramonium* layer, which began as a reaction to the abuse, predisposed her to a host of other illnesses and to the next layer. The first remedy given was able to deal with the top layer of pathology but not with the original reason for that layer developing in the first place.

Another effect that can follow abuse is that the girl does not seem able to acknowledge her fear. Instead, for her, sexuality takes on an intense quality. She may have a high sex drive and may masturbate. She becomes sexually promiscuous and there is an edge to this activity that suggests she is deliberately playing with fire. The idea of a sexual rendezvous in some risqué place, on the street, or outside a club, with a stranger who has a rough look about him, can be very stimulating for her. There is nothing soft about such sexuality; her actions or behaviors intimately link her sexuality to her rage, turning this child into a sexual predator.

Here too we find the two sides of *Stramonium.* On the one side is the teenager that, like *Hyoscyamus,* ravages her sexual partner and on the other side is the teenager who is in terror of sex and wants to escape any situation in which she feels any sexual overtones.

# MUSCULOSKELETAL SYSTEM

### Back

Here, the two most interesting indicators for *Stramonium* are related to acute upper respiratory tract infections and to seizures. The seizure activity may bring on an attack in which the back stiffens and arches, sometimes to opisthotonos. For a fuller description, see the *Seizures* portion of the **Nervous System** section.

Upper respiratory tract infections may occasionally be quite severe for the *Stramonium* patient. During such attacks an older child may tell his parent that his back feels cold and that he needs to cover it up. You may even see him shiver. As the infection progresses to a terribly dry, harsh cough, he may strain his muscles or diaphragm. Now he begins to have back pain. Every time he coughs, he feels pain in his back. Later, as the infection continues, the cervical glands enlarge and the sternocleidomastoid contracts, causing pain in the neck. This may even lead to a torticollis in addition to the infection, the dry cough, and the terrible mood. *Lycopodium* may mistakenly be given at this point, as it shares many of these symptoms.

### Extremities

In the extremities, there are three symptoms that *Stramonium* shares with *Medorrhinum*. First is the confusion in sidedness: *Stramonium* may be delayed in deciding whether they are left-handed or right-handed. Secondly, many of the children will bite their nails or pick at their cuticles. Thirdly, many of the children prefer to have their extremities uncovered, even though a subset may have extremities that are cold to the touch.

# FEVER AND CHILLS

*Stramonium* is notable for chills and fever in the materia medica and is also listed strongly in the repertory for both. Mostly, given a choice of the two, it is fever that will present in the majority of the child's complaints. The chills are more likely to accompany an acute infection, usually preceding it. They will be felt most strongly in the back and in the extremities.

The fevers are often so striking that, to the homeopathic prescriber, it is clear that the child needs a remedy which fits the mental and neurologic symptoms, rather than the common symptoms or the modalities of the fever. Fevers accompany many respiratory tract infections and may run quite high. The child may become delirious, not knowing where he is; he may see imaginary things and imaginary people who are trying to do horrible things to him. In this state, the fear may drive him to attempt escape, and in trying to do so, he may become violent and seem like a wild animal. So we see him going from the delirium of the confusion segment into the fear segment and from there into violent overreaction.

During fever, he may bore his head into the pillow or the bed, or have twitches of his face or extremities, or possibly even have a febrile seizure. He may also have a red face, dry mouth, thirst for cold drinks, little urination or stool, photophobia, and headaches.

## STRAMONIUM

Alec's case is a typical example of a fever that is treatable with *Stramonium*. In the middle of a streptococcal infection, five year old Alec developed a very high fever. When his mother went into the room to check on him, she must inadvertently have made a slight noise. He woke up frightened, shrieking that the wallpaper was going to attack him. He also said that someone was pushing him down and keeping him down on the bed. He begged for his mother to come into the room, although she was in the room at the time. He cried that he could not see and wanted his mother to turn on the lights, even though they were already on. He was screaming, "I can't see! I can't see!" He began to scream that there were strings holding him down. His muscles were all taut and tense, his eyes glazed over, his face full of fear. He was talking constantly but not making any sense at all. Alec's fever illustrates a point worth mentioning. The fever, which belongs to the violent overreaction segment of *Stramonium*, is usually associated with the fear segment which also erupts and leads either to violence or to terror.

In general, there is scanty perspiration in *Stramonium*, except during sleep, when it may be quite profuse.

# SKIN

Many of these children may have a skin rash, usually diagnosed as eczema. In such children it is most often allergic in nature, and worsens when the child eats dairy, wheat or citrus. The rash itself is nondescript but treatment of it is seen as paramount. The rash tends to be present more on the left upper side and lower right side; the left hand is a common site. The most likely outcome of taking allopathic medication at this juncture is that, if it is effective and the child gets rid of the eczema, then seizures, tics, fears or other emotional changes will promptly follow.

Such a scenario brings to mind a common route by which the homeopathic prescriber will often come to *Stramonium* as the simillimum. Since many of these children have symptoms of other remedies as well, in the early phase of the disorder it is possible that the full *Stramonium* picture will be unrecognizable. After prescribing some other remedy, such as *Sulphur*, which causes the eczema to disappear, the homeopath may then witness a suppression, in which all of a sudden, the mental/emotional symptoms appear full-blown, presenting a clear picture of the simillimum, *Stramonium*.

*Stramonium* has cured spots and rashes of various diagnoses which are red and itchy and tend to occur over the lower abdomen and groin area, as well as on the buttocks. Likewise, vitiligo, or loss of skin pigment, may sometimes be cured with this remedy. My friend, Vassilis Ghegas MD, made a poetic point in one of his lectures, a point that resonates with my premise of the remedy—that the *Stramonium* child, so full of darkness, may create vitiligo as a compensation, producing white to compensate for the darkness within the child.

Allergic reactions may be seen in hives, especially as a reaction to drugs. While the hives may not be distinctive, the point that most leads one to consider *Stramonium* is that the hive reaction tends to occlude the air passages. As the child begins to choke, a *Stramonium* state begins. After such an episode, the child may end up with chronic allergies, asthma, or neurodermatitis. What is more troubling is that he may also develop fears, ritualistic behaviors, and perhaps violence.

Allergic reactions may also be expressed as a neurodermatitis combined with eczema. The history may be similar to that mentioned above with the eczema. Four year old Roland's story is typical: food allergies, combined with allergy to wool, began his eczema. After the rash covered a great deal of his legs, his parents applied steroids but as the eczema receded, he developed neurodermatitis. He now scratched every part of his body he could reach. His scratching created many cuts all over his body, cuts that allowed staphylococcal and streptococcal impetigo to begin. Roland's parents were discouraged because every episode was more severe than the previous one and with every episode they had to give stronger medicines. They were convinced that this cycle would never end and that Roland would end up in a life threatening situation. They began to use coal tar solutions, steroids, and antibiotics in conjunction to keep the rashes in check. The rashes did not disappear, they were only subdued, and the flare-ups continued. Roland still scratched his face terribly at night, as he was falling asleep and when he woke up, scratching at it as if he were a wild animal. His skin also itched in the bath and so he bathed infrequently.

While Roland's parents were happy that he scratched less than before, they were concerned that his behavior had changed since the rash had decreased in severity. If awakened he would become angry and when angry

## STRAMONIUM

he would scratch himself intensely. If he was tired and wanted something that his parents did not wish to give him, he scratched himself and yelled. He developed nightmares, during which he again scratched himself. Roland had been a pleasant though very clingy baby. He did not like to play with other children or to be left by his parents. He often cried and wanted to be picked up. When he was six months old his mother had to be away from home for two weeks, because she was caring for her dying mother. It was then that the eczema and noticeable allergies began.

I gave Roland one dose of *Stramonium* 200C. In just three weeks, his rash was mostly gone, his emotions were less likely to flare up, his scratching was minimal and he became more social, no longer wanting to stay at home. He made friends and was playing well. A five month follow-up showed Roland feeling well. By then he was off all his skin medicines, had no flare-ups and was well emotionally.

I would like to end Roland's description with an observation I made while watching Roland scratch his face and eyes. It looked to me like a movie in which the character was so beset by grief that he tore at his face and ripped his eyes out. Whenever Roland would finish scratching, or rather, when his mother finally could hold his hands down, his face would be marked with tracks of bleeding cuts, as if an animal paw had just clawed at his face. The impression I was left with was a boy who was frightened to be alone without his parents and who, when his mother left him for two weeks, felt such a strong shock that allergies kicked in and eventually drove him to aggressively attack his own body. It was as if all the terror and violence that *Stramonium* can produce was aimed at himself.

## NERVOUS SYSTEM

Symptoms within the nervous system can be categorized as follows:
1) True seizures
2) Athetoid motions
3) Jerking motions
4) General etiology
5) Meningitis, both as specific etiology and as treatment for the disease

## Seizures

Epilepsy, with or without an abnormal EEG, has been treated with and cured by *Stramonium*. The seizures are varied, but do have some common features. *Stramonium* is one of the most common remedies for febrile seizures. It may be the indicated remedy for children whose seizures occur more frequently when they are overheated or during/after a hot shower. Another common characteristic I have found is that most of the EEG findings are on the left side, as if injuries to the left side of the head were more likely to put someone into a *Stramonium* state. Yet another common characteristic, though not universally found in *Stramonium* children, is that the child maintains consciousness during the attack.

Some *Stramonium* seizures can be so mild that they resemble the shivering and teeth chattering that go with chilliness. Such mild seizures could be petit mal or absence seizures. They may also resemble some descriptions of night terrors. For example, Lorraine describes a seizure experienced by her eleven year old daughter. "There we are driving along and all of a sudden Nancy begins to moan. Then she gets this staring look, like she sees me but is looking right through me, like she doesn't recognize me, and she starts to scream, 'The monsters are after me. Get them away from me! Hug me! Hug me! Hold me!' When I later asked Nancy about it, she told me, 'The monsters are weird, like a nightmare.'"

Fifteen year old Alan's description of what he experiences sheds further light on these nightmarish episodes. "They are out of a dream, or connected to a dream. A lot of times just before they come on, I get this feeling like I've experienced it before, right out of a dream I had last night. Pretty soon after that I'm in the middle of the attack."

Others further describe the attacks. "I stay awake during it, I know it is happening. In fact I am so aware that I try to bluff my way through it, you know, like I stumble, but keep on walking so that I won't look like a jerk."

Another child has his seizures during the night. When the parents hear strange noises they run into the room. The child says to them, during the attack, "I'm having another one," as he jerks to one side while his arms flail to the other.

In a sense, this activity shows the relevance of the well-known rubric for *Stramonium*: **Convulsions, with consciousness.** The effect seen is very similar to night terrors, in which the alive conscious side is frightened (thus overcontrolled), while the demonic unconscious side, with its convulsions and contortions, seems possessed. **The 'fight or flight' response is engaged and the *Stramonium* child's two poles grow even further apart.**

In other cases, the seizures may look shockingly severe as with tonic clonic seizures. As mentioned before, the individual may be conscious during these seizures. But, unlike the mild attacks previously described, these have a great deal of commotion associated with them. The child may smile or the jaw may move up and down, as if he is chewing, clenching or talking. Yet he will be unable to answer. One may observe a Jacksonian march, in which the convulsion begins at the foot or hand and moves upwards. The eyes may be wide open or may blink, distort, or roll. The head will move to one side or jerk from one side to the other. The neck may be drawn sideways or the child may progress into opisthotonos, with clenched fingers and thumbs. Temporal lobe epilepsy fits this remedy as well.

Ryan's attacks are an example of the more severe type. Soon after a DPT vaccination, at the age of one year, Ryan began to have seizures. These were first diagnosed as benign infantile spasms and later as focal seizures. They were originally mild. Ryan would stare straight ahead and occasionally become stiff in his extremities. Eventually he came to have six to twenty attacks a day. They would begin with a look of fear on his face, accompanied by shrieking, after which he would 'freak out' in front of his family. He would try to run to his mother's lap, his arms and legs would twitch, and he would develop myoclonus. While becoming rigid, he would jerk his arms and head, and tilt his head to one side, his face reddening. Eventually he was diagnosed with generalized clonic seizures; they could not be controlled by any medicines. At this same time, he also experienced night terrors, began grinding his teeth at night and dreaming of witches, along with developing many other fears common to the remedy.

In most children who have seizures and need *Stramonium*, the vivid personality will clearly indicate this remedy; the homeopath will rarely have to decide based solely on the seizure symptoms. At one extreme of the picture, for example, there is Sally, a five year old, who shows the introverted side of *Stramonium*. Tending most of the time to whisper when she speaks, she is too timid to play with others. During the seizures, however, she becomes downright violent, scratching and tearing at people. On the other side of the spectrum is Alice, who is fourteen years old. The first time I saw her she was wearing all black and had tattoos on her arms and forearms. She loved to read novels about the devil and about ghosts. So, at one extreme we have a girl who is struggling to be the perfect, good child, and suffers from her own over-control, while on the other we have a girl who has slid into a hellish environment and finds it hideously enjoyable. Again, the two prominent poles repeat themselves even in this disease.

## Athetoid Motion

You may, on occasion, see a slightly autistic child with pervasive developmental delay and perhaps some violence, who exhibits involuntary motions. In a child that shows only these, you would think first of *Hyoscyamus*, but if the child is violent and, in addition, fearful, *Stramonium* should take the lead. For example, you may find a two year old *Stramonium* child moving his left hand and arm in a choreic, involuntary circle in front of his face, almost as if the hand is moving by itself. The circle starts out wide and then contracts tighter and tighter into smaller circles. All this happens, seemingly unbeknownst to the child, while he is tearing up his book or throwing things around the room. In another case, one eye closes, then both eyes close, then they both open. Staring right through the doctor, the child starts laughing at some gruesome joke known only to him.

If you have a rocking chair or rocking horse in your office, you may observe the child convulsively rocking his whole body on it, hard and fast, arching his back, looking up at the ceiling, then down at the floor, then up at the ceiling, back and forth, violently, a behavior you may also observe in *Tarentula hispanica*. He is laughing and making guttural sounds and rolling his head from side to side, as his arms flail around without his control.

He may do all sorts of things with his hands. The hands are the most mobile part of the body during these involuntary actions. One moment, both hands are up in front of the face with bent wrists, looking like a praying mantis. Next, they are moving clockwise or counterclockwise from the wrist. Still later, his hands may hang limply by his side, or his arms will be outstretched above him, and then his hands hide his face until they again begin to move. The child loses control of his arms, moving them involuntarily and gracefully, as if swimming.

# STRAMONIUM

The child's gait may be funny or odd in appearance, whether wide, unsteady, falling, or ataxic. Occasionally he may walk only on the balls of his feet, never letting his heels touch the ground. This is neurologic in nature, for the muscles and bones are all well. Significantly, the oddness of this gait increases as the child becomes more and more excited.

## Jerking Motions

Some of the jerking motions occur while the child is stammering. At the same time, the eyes may blink a lot. If the stammer is intense, there may be twitching in the face or even jerking motions of the arms.

There may also be involuntary motion in the diaphragm. In such cases, the child will constantly suck up air, in and out, very loudly and forcibly.

Involuntary jerking of the head off the pillow, after lying down to rest, may be seen. As discussed in the **Head** section, as well as in the *Meningitis* subsection following, this symptom is mostly observed during infections and fevers.

Another behavior which is very similar to that of *Hyoscyamus*, can be seen in the child who, when frightened, may jump up and grab hold of his penis.

Gilles de la Tourette's syndrome may be ameliorated by the use of this remedy. Symptoms can begin in childhood, around seven to eleven years, with multiple tics anywhere in the body. By the time the individual enters puberty, however, the facial tics, echolalia (involuntary repetition of words that are heard), cursing and involuntary barking may already have begun, as well as the tendency to hold his penis. All these symptoms will be very similar to *Hyoscyamus*. Yet if violence is present along with fears, accompanied by intense facial expressions when vocalizing, this would indicate *Stramonium*. Besides tics and echolalia there may be uncontrolled motions, including hitting himself or banging his head on the ground. Also similar to *Hyoscyamus*, the child will automatically voice aloud any thought that occurs to him, without any intervening filter. Another clue pointing to the need for this remedy is that the *Stramonium* pathology and etiology will often be present even before the onset of the Tourette's. In such cases, the only point that could cause confusion in finding the remedy would be from focusing too much on the symptoms that are common to this disorder, as opposed to focusing on those that most represent the individual.

BODY

## Etiology

The etiology for nervous system disorders includes injuries to the brain, meningitis, fevers and other infections that affect the brain, bad effects from vaccinations, suppressed skin eruptions, and birth traumas. For instance, a head injury received in a car accident, followed by a major personality change in which the person comes to exist only in a world of evil, would fit *Stramonium*.

Frights are one of the most common triggers for seizure disorders in *Stramonium*. Frights from masks, from being forced to be alone, or being attacked by an animal, can all cause the seizure. We have treated several children who developed their first seizure when being forced to go into water. For instance, the child screams that he does not want a bath, and, on being forced into the water, he has a seizure. Similarly, if the child does not wish to learn how to swim but is thrown into the water, he may have his first seizure soon after.

## Meningitis

Although meningitis is one etiology for bringing about a *Stramonium* state, it is also a good remedy to think of *during* the infection itself. In some cases, it can result from a poorly treated ear infection which is allowed to continue until a frank meningitis presents. Surgery can also be responsible for the onset of meningitis. For example, Nicholas has been a terror for several years now, yet prior to this time he had been a very mild child. In search of an etiology, I found that, after having surgery to correct his strabismus, he had developed bacterial meningitis. The change in behavior followed that infection.

During an infection, the child may undergo fits of unconsciousness, at times entering delirium, followed by a return to consciousness. Often there is a progression from chills, through fever, to vomiting, headache and finally, convulsions. Early on, the eyes and ears can become sensitive to both light and noise. The forehead may wrinkle. The child then becomes sleepless and delirious, exhibiting a combination of fear and violence. His eyes will be wide open, staring out. His lips and jaw may move back and forth, as if speaking. In an attempt to push away that which is frightening him, he may begin to scream, hit, or bite. He will often fear shiny objects or glasses of water. In fact, he may fear water in general. During the delirium he may also hold his genitals, as does *Hyoscyamus*.

As in *Helleborus*, the child may burrow his head into the pillow and grind his teeth during the stupor. In addition, the following *Stramonium* keynote may be present: raising the head off the bedding every so often. While no one is sure why *Stramonium* does this, upon observing some of these children and adults during such behavior, the impression the observer is left with is that they are trying to fight off sleep. It looks like a tactic they use to stay awake, in their attempt to avoid facing all the horror that they will meet, once again, in sleep. Lifting the head up from the pillow, with a jerking motion seems to say, "Oh my God, I almost fell asleep."

Luke exemplifies the *Stramonium* encephalitis. He was five years old when the infection began, initially a streptococcal infection treated with antibiotics. Soon afterwards, he became very dizzy and lethargic. Within one week, he could not be awakened in the morning very easily. That morning, while showering, he had a seizure. His parents tried to talk to him but he would not answer. That day, he was sitting in a chair and just slid right out of it. His eyes rolled up, his head jerked backwards, and he became unconscious. He was rushed to the emergency room in a status epilepticus and placed on massive doses of medication to lessen the attack. He slipped in and out of a coma for weeks.

Since that time, two years ago, his personality has changed markedly. Whereas he used to be a sweet boy, now he has become angry and aggressive. He kicks, spits, bites, pulls hair, and has night terrors in which his eyes acquire a glare and a far-off look, like "some kind of sadist". His intelligence has dropped; although he had been able to learn easily before, he can now learn things only with difficulty. He used to be bright and sociable; now he is averse to people and to groups. He still has many seizures each day. At night, he has night terrors of the devil or believes that he will die soon. *Stramonium* reversed this personality change, bringing him back to his old self, as well as decreasing the seizures.

BODY

# MOTHER, FATHER, PREGNANCY, and NEWBORN

**The state of the mother before or during pregnancy may have predisposed the child to need *Stramonium* for two different reasons. First, it is possible that it was the mother who initially needed the *Stramonium*.** For instance, there may be a history of encephalitis in the mother a few years before or during the pregnancy. The mother may seem to have recovered, yet the baby may have needed *Stramonium* ever since the very start of his life. It would appear that any illness involving the possibility either of brain injury or of central nervous system dysfunction in the mother can, in turn, send the infant into a *Stramonium* state. Infections to the central nervous system, kidney diseases that affect the brain, such as pyelonephritis or renal failure, or fevers that affect the brain may all, during pregnancy, be an etiology for *Stramonium* in the mother and then in the child.

**Secondly, frights during pregnancy may affect the child and cause him to become *Stramonium*.** In such a situation, the mother may not have become a *Stramonium*, even though she did experience the fright. For example, she could have been a *Calcarea carbonica* and experienced the fright in the way a *Calcarea carbonica* would. However, when the baby is born it needs *Stramonium*, as if it too, experienced the fright, or at least felt the mother's reaction to the fright, and responded by becoming *Stramonium*. Typically in this situation the mother will maintain that reaction (that *Stramonium* fear) as long as she is pregnant. After labor that particular fear may be gone, yet it will still be found in the baby.

Having observed this often enough over the years, I have taken to thinking that if the fetus can experience the mother's reaction to that fear, why is it not possible for the mother to continue to experience the child's reaction to her initial reaction? Thus, for the remaining portion of her pregnancy she feels these fears, but after the birth, the baby as well as his reactions are now outside the mother's body and so she is no longer feeling it. It is interesting to find that the child will be frightened by the same thing (be it noise or water or certain types of people) that caused the initial fright during pregnancy. Even more interesting is that the child may not have been told of the mother's fright and yet will respond to the same situation in very much the same way as the mother did.

# STRAMONIUM

It is also sometimes found that due to a fright that the mother suffered, or due to illness (even if it was only severe nausea and vomiting), **the baby was almost miscarried during the first trimester.**

Other problems can arise from **complications during labor or birth, which separate the mother from the baby and prevent them from bonding.** The abandonment issue may possibly begin then, when the baby is left alone in the hospital.

Sometimes an infant will be born extremely underweight, seemingly malnourished. He may appear frightened and hungry or exhibit transient tachypnea, as does *Aconitum napellus*. It is also possible that the infant was delivered in a quick labor—as Lucretius put it, "Thrown up like a sailor from the cruel wave...onto the shores of light,"—with the umbilical cord wrapped around his neck and/or that the head was bruised.

Alternately, the mother may say that it was a difficult birth, lasting several days, finally requiring vacuum extraction, and that the child was delivered with a low pulse, with little tone of body, and a diagnosis of a subarachnoid hemorrhage. Soon afterwards, a further diagnosis may be made, such as cerebral palsy or occasional seizures.

A common story for *Stramonium* infants is that of repeated colds, bronchitis, ear infections, and a tendency towards loose stools. They may develop eczema within the first two months. This eczema, if treated, may disappear after several months, only to be followed by asthma at about one year and violence and fears by eighteen months.

**Turning to the father, we may find that he tends to have strong emotional outbursts, or a history of a nervous breakdown. This might also be present among the father's siblings. Strongly characteristic for these violent fathers is a history of alcoholism, perhaps over several generations.** In addition, the father may either be missing, or working too much, so that he is not present in the child's life. The father may also dislike, or be distant toward the child. In all of these instances, what the child experiences is a frightening sense of loss or isolation.

BODY

# PHYSICAL GENERAL SYMPTOMS

*Stramonium* has not been known for the presence of any common characteristic physical symptoms. However, I have so frequently observed the symptoms listed below that I often use them to confirm the remedy, especially if, in a differential diagnosis of the case, *Stramonium* is close to another remedy.

In spite of the fact that the vast majority of these children are either warm-blooded or have chilly parts to their body, they appear to be **aggravated by the heat.** They act out more, are more restless, suffer sunstroke and seizures, and sleep more poorly in the heat. They may like being in cold water, like *Medorrhinum.*

I would say it is fairly characteristic of *Stramonium* that they **do not like some aspect of the sun;** either they will complain of the heat, or that the light hurts their eyes, or they become fearful from the glare.

A very strong feature that I have found in many *Stramonium* children and adults is that the symptoms of the eyes, ears, and nose may be on the left side, but, as the symptoms are viewed in descending order down the body, they become more characteristically right-sided. *Stramonium* is listed in the repertory in plain type in the rubric: **GENERALITIES: Crosswise, left upper and right lower.** I believe it should be elevated to italics, as I consider this to be a very reliable symptom. It should also be added to the rubric: **GENERALITIES: Side, left.**

**General aggravations in the dark or during sleep** are common, as described throughout the book. For some children, **midnight and 2 a.m. constitute strong aggravation times.** Although seizures may occur during this time frame, restless sleep, headaches, and night terrors are more common.

**Wind and rain** may aggravate the child. Many of these children will be frightened by the wind as it seems to cause such turmoil in the trees all around them. This is especially true of the fearful child. However, if the child has come to be more aggressive and perhaps somewhat demonic, he may instead positively enjoy the wind and rain, even feeling his best when an electric storm moves through the area.

These children may have **high energy all day** and never experience any down time. Or they may nap for a short period of time in the afternoon, thus enabling them to stay up late. Nevertheless, they are **aggravated by missing their sleep** and tend to misbehave much more if not well-rested.

**Sweets** tend to make the child more hyperactive or violent, while **milk** and **smoke** tend to aggravate the asthma and respiratory tract infections.

The children may show the famous keynote of *Stramonium*, **Painlessness of complaints.** In a way, it is fitting for this type of child, who acts as if he were already dead, not to feel pain. The introverted, hypervigilant subtype, however, will naturally feel pain and may actually be hypersensitive to it.

Over three hundred and fifty cases comprise the material for this **monograph,** and, of these individuals, **many began to exhibit symptoms of the remedy at around two years of age.** Perhaps this is the age at which the child first clearly perceives that he is different from his parents, separate in some way. While this is the normal developmental stage for the two year old to begin experiencing *some* fear, it is also true that specific events during this particular stage seem most likely to predispose him to the development of the *Stramonium* picture. In light of this, I often instruct the parents of my youngest patients to make sure as much as is feasible to shield the child from any possible frights that may trigger the development of this picture.

# ETIOLOGY

**Bad reactions to vaccinations** occur in many *Stramonium* infants. Some will have seizures, others high fever, or both combined, and most will scream for extended periods of time. During such a time, they may have trouble sleeping, drifting into sleep for only short naps and waking as if from fright. Some will seem to lose mental ability after any of the vaccinations, though most especially after the DPT vaccine.

While asking one mother about allergies she said, "Why yes, my son does have allergies, especially to the DPT vaccination. After it, he began to vomit, had seizures and high fevers, and stopped eating for two weeks."

An **etiology of fright** is very common in *Stramonium*. Two more examples: One mother recounted a story about her son when he was two years old. On the eve of Halloween, a woman friend came to the door dressed as an ugly witch with a mask and big black cape. She came in and called Johnny by name and let out a cackling laugh. He screamed and screamed for several hours and cried himself to sleep. He could not be quieted down. He began to be fearful and hyperactive after this event.

Another child was frightened when he saw his father physically abuse his mother. Fearful ever since, it was also after this that the monster in him had arisen.

**Suppression of skin eruptions is a possible etiology for *Stramonium*.** The child's history will show that eczema and other skin rashes were treated, and as the rash receded, the *Stramonium* picture developed.

**Surgery itself, along with the anesthesia and staying in the hospital surrounded by strangers, seems to send some children into *Stramonium*.** For example, one boy had to have bladder surgery; within two months after the operation, he developed night terrors, fears, and twitching. Another boy had surgery to correct his strabismus. Two months after the surgery he developed meningitis and became both hyperactive and violent, and remained in that state for several years until receiving *Stramonium*.

**Another etiology is physical shock from injury.** The injury may be so severe or the child's reaction to the pain so extreme that he enters the *Stramonium* fright, and in time the full picture emerges, brought about by the sheer amount of pain. He acts as if he is being tortured. In addition, the child may have to undergo a medical procedure (to correct the injury) without understanding it and perhaps without the parents even being present. Again, isolation mingled with pain and fear is the outcome.

The pattern of shock, injury and abandonment, all too common in the *Stramonium* history, is experienced by the child who has been repeatedly beaten by the parent. The parent may later give him the cold shoulder, or refuse to talk to him or, even worse, leave him or give him away. These same emotions may be felt by the child who has been taken away from the birth parents and placed in another situation. **Thus we see that at the root of many *Stramonium* cases is a feeling of aloneness and a lack of protection. The child, not surprisingly, feels abandoned to some monster that is about to eat him up.**

# Appendix

# Appendix

# *Aphorisms*

A short guided tour through the aphorisms of the Organon which most emphatically illustrate the process of vitalistic homeopathic practice.

**Aphorisms 9 and 10 tell us that the vital force is within us, animating us.**

> # 9: In the state of health, the vital force animating the material human organism reigns in supreme sovereignty. It maintains the sensations and activities of all the parts of the living organism in a harmony that obliges wonderment. The reasoning vital force, who inhabits the organism can thus freely use this healthy living instrument to reach the lofty goal of human existence.

> #10: Without the vital force, the material organism is unable to feel, or act, or maintain itself. Only because of the immaterial vital force that animates it in health and in disease can it feel and maintain its vital functions.

**Aphorism 22 explains how and why the vital force maintains a balance in us and why it fails when a stress comes.**

> #22: …The vital force was given to us, to sustain our life in harmony as long as we are healthy, not to heal itself when diseased, for if it possessed an ability so worthy of imitation, it would never allow the organism to fall ill. When afflicted by disease agents, our vital force can express its untunement only through disturbances in the normal functions of the organism and through pain, whereby it calls for the help of a wise physician.

**Aphorism 16 says that when a big enough stress affects the vital force, the vital force strains and we become ill.**

> # 16: Outer malefic agents that harm the healthy organism and disturb the harmonious rhythm of life can reach and affect the vital force only in a way that also is dynamic and vital….

# STRAMONIUM

**Aphorisms 11 and 12 further clarify that when we become ill it is the vital force that first is ill.**

#11: When man falls ill, at first it is only this self-sustaining vital force everywhere present in the organism which is untuned by the dynamic influence of the hostile disease agent....

#12: It is only the pathologically untuned vital force that causes diseases.

**Aphorisms 11 and 14 show that the strained vital force is what produces symptoms that we call disease.**

# 11: ...It is only this vital force thus untuned which brings about in the organism the disagreeable sensations and abnormal functions that we call disease.

#14: There is no curable disease or morbific alteration hidden in the interior of the body which does not announce itself to the conscientiously observant physician through objective and subjective symptoms....

**If everything quoted is true so far, then it follows that disease is a totality and that all symptoms show *the totality of the strain* of the vital force. Aphorisms 6, 7, and 18 demonstrate this point.**

# 6: ...he sees in any given case of disease only the disturbance of the body and soul which are perceptible to the senses: subjective symptoms, incidental symptoms, objective symptoms, i.e., deviations from the former healthy condition of the individual now sick which the patient personally feels, which people around him notice, which the physician sees in him.

The totality of these perceptible signs represent the entire extent of the sickness; together they constitute its true and only conceivable form.

# 7: ...So it is the totality of symptoms, the outer image expressing the inner essence of the disease, i.e., of the disturbed vital force, that must be the main, even the only means by which the disease allows us to find the necessary remedy...Briefly, in every individual case of disease the totality of the symptoms must be the physician's principal concern, the only object of his attention....

# 18: It is an indubitable truth that there is nothing else but the

totality of symptoms—including the concomitant circumstances of the case by which a disease can express its need for help.

**Therefore, when stress affects the vital force, the vital force strains and becomes ill, creating and pouring out symptoms that show the strain, which we call disease. The disease then is in the functioning of the vital force; the symptoms are the representation, the effect, of the disease. This is the essence of aphorism 15.**

> #15: In the invisible interior of the body, the suffering of the pathologically untuned vital force animating the organism and the totality of the perceptible symptoms that result and that represent the disease are one and the same.
>
> The organism is the material instrument of life; but it is no more conceivable without the life-giving, regulating, instinctively feeling vital force than this vital force is conceivable without the organism. The two are one, even if thought separates them to facilitate comprehension.

**This means that when we treat with homeopathy, we are working by treating the vital force, as described in aphorisms 16 and 19.**

> #16: …The physician can remove these pathological untunements (diseases) only by acting on our vital force… So it is by the dynamic action upon the vital force that remedies can restore health and the harmony of life….

> # 19: Since diseases are only deviations from the healthy condition, and since they express themselves through symptoms, and since cure is equally only a change from the diseased condition back to the state of health, one easily sees that medicines can cure disease only if they possess the power to alter the way a person feels and functions. Indeed, it is only because of this power that they are medicines.

# STRAMONIUM

**By observation, Hahnemann found that diseases that are similar to each other cure or cancel each other out, as in aphorisms 25, 26, 27.**

#25: …the medicine that has produced upon a healthy human body the greatest number of symptoms similar to those of the disease being treated is the only one that will cure… All medicines without exception cure those diseases whose symptoms most closely resemble their own, and leave none of them uncured.

#26: …In the living organism a weaker dynamic affection is permanently extinguished by a stronger one, which, though different in nature, nevertheless greatly resembles it in expression.

#27: The curative virtue of medicines thus depends on the symptoms being similar to those of the disease, but stronger.

**We choose remedies that act on healthy people in toxic doses similar to the way the disease acts on sick people, as in aphorisms 18, 24, 27, 29.**

#18: …We can categorically declare that the totality of symptoms and circumstances observed in each individual case is the one and only indication that can guide us to the choice of the remedy.

#24: …This therapy chooses from among all the remedies whose actions upon the healthy have been established that one which has the power and propensity to produce an artificial disease condition most similar to the natural one being treated. This remedy is used for the totality of symptoms of a case….

#27: …It follows that in any particular case, a disease can be destroyed and removed most surely, thoroughly, swiftly, and permanently only by a medicine that can make a human being feel a totality of symptoms most completely similar to it but stronger.

#29: Any disease that is not exclusively a surgical case consists of a particular pathological, dynamic untunement of feelings and functions in our vital force.

So in homeopathic cure this vital force, which has been dynamically untuned by natural disease, is taken over by a similar and somewhat stronger artificial disease, through the administration of a potentized medicine that has been accurately chosen for the similarity of its symptoms.

Consequently the weaker natural dynamic disease is extinguished and disappears, from then on it no longer exists for the vital force, which is controlled and occupied only by the stronger artificial disease; this in turn presently wanes, so that the patient is left free and cured. Thus…the vital force can again maintain the organism in health.

**This means that, when we treat someone and cure them, we will see the symptoms disappear, as in aphorisms 8, 12, and 22.**

> # 8: After the elimination of all the symptoms and perceptible signs of disease, one cannot imagine or demonstrate by any experiment in the world that anything but health remains, that anything but health can remain….
>
> # 12: …Conversely, the cessation through treatment of all the symptoms, i.e., the disappearance of all perceptible deviations from health, necessarily implies that the vital force has recovered its integrity and therefore that the whole organism has returned to health.
>
> # 22: To change diseases into health the only thing that must be removed is the totality of the subjective and objective symptoms.

**That cure is the total successful treatment of the total disease, as in aphorisms 7, 16, 17.**

> # 7: …Briefly, in every individual case of disease the totality of the symptoms must be the physician's principal concern, the only object of his attention, the only thing to be removed by his intervention in order to cure, i.e., to transform the disease into health.
>
> # 16: …So it is by the dynamic action upon the vital force that remedies can restore health and the harmony of life after the perceptible changes in health (the totality of symptoms) have revealed the disease to the carefully observing and inquiring physician fully enough to be cured.
>
> # 17: Cure which is the elimination of all the perceptible signs and symptoms of disease, means also the removal of the inner modifications of the vital force which underlie them: in this way the whole disease has been destroyed.
>
> Consequently the physician has only to eliminate the totality of

## STRAMONIUM

symptoms in order to remove simultaneously the inner alteration, the pathological untunement of the vital force, thereby entirely removing and annihilating the disease itself.

# The New England School of Homeopathy

The New England School of Homeopathy (NESH) was created in 1987 to translate homeopathic philosophy into the successful and predictable practice of medicine. Our goal is for practitioners of homeopathy to fulfill their potential role in health care—to help people attain freedom from illness on the mental, emotional, and physical planes so they may better realize their highest aspirations.

**To fulfill this mission, the program and materials of NESH strive:**
- To exemplify the highest purpose and achievement in the field of homeopathic medicine. NESH aims to inspire the greater homeopathic community to join in this endeavor, and to encourage and assist the non-homeopathic community in the exploration of and participation in homeopathy.
- To commit the full energies of NESH to provide each participant with the tools required for the successful practice of homeopathy in a thorough and expedient manner.
- To provide a philosophical foundation based on the principles of classical homeopathy.
- To establish a practical technical foundation essential to the successful practice of homeopathy.
- To transform homeopathic theory into predictable clinical results.
- To provide materials which are clinically significant and immediately applicable.
- To communicate actual experience. All materials bearing the NESH name have been clinically verified by the presenter.

## The vehicles for accomplishment of these objectives are:

- Professional classes designed:
    - to educate the beginning practitioner in the effective application of homeopathy.
    - to enhance the practicing homeopath's knowledge, so that he or she may deliver consistently favorable results.
    - to foster the acquisition of techniques which will enable the practitioner to continue to learn from his/her own experience.
- A journal through which practitioners may learn and share their own discoveries with the homeopathic community. The journal serves to express a shared vision and create a resource for optimal learning by practitioners of all levels.
- A clinical setting for practitioners to support the transition from student to practicing clinician.
- An ongoing forum offering participants the opportunity to make the transition from clinician to teacher.
- Seminars presented by clinicians with expertise in a specialized area of homeopathy.
- Publication of reference texts which are relevant for the continuing education of homeopathic physicians and patients.
- Classes for the community at large which illuminate homeopathic theory and application, and encourage the growth of a patient population that is well-educated in the practice of homeopathy.

*For more information write to:*

New England School of Homeopathy
356 Middle Street
Amherst, Massachusetts 01002
(413) 253-5949 • Fax: (413) 256-6223
www.nesh.com • nesh@nesh.com

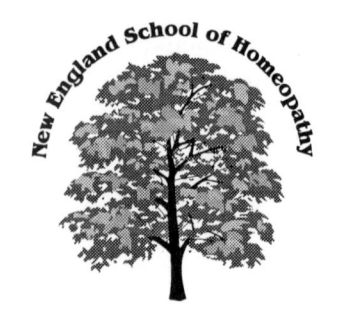

# Index

Abandonment and birth process, 56
Abandonment in hospital at birth and *Stramonium* state, 174
Abandonment, 29, 33, 60, 62, 70, 125, 126, 132, 145, 154, 166
Abdomen, 157-158
Abdomen, sleeping on, 132
Abdominal complaints and somatized fear, 158
Abdominal pain, xi, 12
Absence seizures, 167
Abuse by child, 71
Abuse predisposes her to other illnesses, 162
Abuse real or impression of by parents during night terror, 125
Abuse, 61, 99, 101, 120, 145
Abuse, sexual, 61, 161
Abusive to others without fear of punishment, 84
Accidents, dream of, 66
*Aconitum napellus*, 174
Act, desire to, 30
Acting out world view, 20
Acting out, 19, 34, 44, 47, 49, 78, 84, 101, 103, 158
Acute ear infection, 142
Acute illness, 38
Acute infection preceding chills, 163
Acute pathologic states, 15
Acute states and permanent states from fear, 45
Addictive quality of violence, 80
Addiction loop and systems dynamics, 65
Admonished, will weep when, 85
Aether, 3
Affection withheld as control mechanism, 72
After death, question of living again, 51
After effects of ear infection, 142
Ages 3-6 for start of Landau-Kleffner syndrome, 113
Ages 7 or 8 using sexual language, 160
Aggression and shyness in *Medorrhinum*, 43
Aggression, mimicked, 79
Aggression, 43, 66, 89, 92-93, 105, 175
Air passages occluded in hives reaction, 165
Air, sucking, loudly and forcibly, 170
Airborne allergy, 151
Air travel, 58-59
Airplanes, sound of, 65
Aisle seat, desires, 13

Alcohol related illness, 69
Alcohol, desire for, 157
Alcoholism of father, 174
Allergies and DPT vaccine, 176
Allergies and chafed, red skin, 148
Allergic hives, as drug reaction, 165
Allergies, 151
Allopathy for rashes and emotional/ physical consequences, 164
Allopathy and asthma, 154
Alone in dreams, 124
Alone, 27, 28, 30, 66, 116, 177
Alone, desire to be, 33 143
Alone, fear of being, xiii, 46, 54, 60
Altered perceptions, 113
*Anacardium*, 16
Anaphylactic shock after antibiotics, 149
Anesthesia as etiology, 177
Angel-like during infections, 154
Anger, 23, 72, 91
Anger and aggression from encephalitis, 172
Anguish, 150
Animal dander aggravates asthma, 153
Animal nature, 34
Animals in dreams, 121
Animals named to ameliorate fear 141
Animals, 57, 70, 125
Animals, fear of, 53, 54, 59
Animals, mean to or tortured, 80, 153
Animals, stuffed, 83
Animals, wild, delusion of in fever, 163
Answer, inability to, in encephalitis, 172
Answers incoherently, 97
Antibiotics and asthma, 153
Antibiotics and autism, 112
Antibiotics and encephalitis, 172
Antibiotics in impetigo, 165
Antibiotics, 152
Antibiotics, severe allergic reaction to, 160
Antibiotics, throat closing after, 149
Antipathic treatments, 155
Anuria, 159
Anus red and sore, 158
Anxiety of day surfaces at night, 116
Anxiety, 122, 125, 148, 158
Aphorisms of Organon, (numbers 6, 7, 8, 9, 10, 11, 12, 14, 15, 16, 17, 18, 19, 22, 24, 25, 27, 29), 181-186
*Apis mellifica*, 159

Apologizes, 71
Appetency, 105
Appetite increased and decreased in *Stramonium*, 155-157
Appetite loss, 152
Appetite returns after remedy, 156
Appetite wanting with thirst, 157
Appetite, 67, 155-157
Apple juice, craves, 156
Approach, fear of, 48, 55
*Argentum nitricum* and *Stramonium* compared, 52
Arguing, 66
Arms flail to one side, child jerks to other in seizures, 167
Arms, jerking motions, 170
*Arnica montana*, 16, 48
*Arnica montana*, in miscarriage, 11
Arrogance, 73, 81, 84
*Arsenicum album*, 143
Arthritis, 23
Ashen face, 147
Asphyxiation, from fear in, as etiology, 154
Associating violence and fear with *Stramonium* incorrectly, 38
Asthma as life threatening disease, 155
Asthma with eczema, 51
Asthma, 51, 73, 74, 153-155, 165
Ataxic gait, 170
Athetoid motions, 169-170
Attack by animals and seizures, 171
Attacked, 75
Attention difficulties and violent manifestations, 92
Attention difficulties, 15, 89-98, 142, 156, 157
Attention span diminished, 98, 152-153
Attention, for only one thing, 98
Attitude, far away, 75
Auditory integration in brain, 145
Aura before seizures, 138
Autism after head injuries, 135
Autism and desire for darkness, 60
Autism and pregnancy, 107
Autism as protective mechanism, 106
Autism, 37, 45, 46, 47, 61, 63, 75, 79, 96, 98, 100, 105-114, 169
Autism, as shutting down, 31
Autistic stare, 139
Auto accident, 135

Automatic behavior, 45, 48, 73, 74
Awakening anxiously, 125
Awareness, lack of, 81

Babbling, 81, 83
Baby dumped out of cradle, 85
Back drawn backwards in seizures, 138
Back, 162-163
Back, cold, in respiratory infection, 162
Back, pain, in respiratory infection, 162
Bacteria, 3
Bacterial meningitis, 76, 171
Bad people, obsessed with, 78
Balance of the conscious and unconscious, 19
Balance of vital force re-established, 8
  See also Aphorisms
Balance, loss of, 57, 64
Balance, precarious, of life and death wish, 32
Balancing act of vital force, 9
Balanitis, 160
Balconies, fright on, 56
Banging his head in Tourette's syndrome, 170
Barking cough, 151
Barking, involuntary, in Tourette's syndrome, 170
*Baryta carbonica*, 160
*Baryta carbonica* and *Helleborus* similarity, 20
*Baryta carbonica* and *Stramonium* compared, 20, 48, 65-66
Basements, dark, fear of, 59, 66, 67
Bathing and bleeding, 11
Bathing and seizures, 171
Bathing and temper tantrums, 51
Bathing, aversion to, yet neat, 153
Bathing, fear of, 112, 119
Bathroom, locked in, panic from, 62, 74
Bathtubs, 65, 141
Bats, fear of 53
Battle field of conscious and unconscious, 32
Battle of wills, 92
Bearded men, 50, 52
Bears, 53, 66
Beast, fierce, like a, going for the kill, 148
Beaten in ear and head, as if, 145
Beaten, fear of being, 116
Bed wetting and fear of water, 127
Bed wetting and night terrors, 126-127
Bed wetting in infection, 149

Bed wetting until late age, 132
Bed, hiding under, 50, 63, 71
Bedroom, own, quality time in, 119
Bedtime, 58
Bedtime, shrieking at, remedies for, 117
Beer, craves, even in three year olds, 157
Begging and pleading, 79, 93, 164
Begs for hugs, 71
*Belladonna*, 136, 137, 143, 147-148, 149, 151-152
Berserk reaction to pets, 54
Birth canal, stuck in, as etiology, 107
Birth canal, 56
Birth process, 56
Birth trauma and eye problems, 140
Birth trauma, 109
Birth traumas as etiology in nervous system disorders, 171
Birth, into brightly lit world, 56
Bites, 71, 73, 74, 78, 79, 80, 92, 172
Biting in headache, 136
Bitten, fear of being, 53, 75
Black and white issues, 112
Black animals, fear of, 53
Black animals, sees, 153
Black cough, global term for whooping cough, 150
Black dogs, 54
Black, wearing all, 169
Blackness, 31
Blame, self, 55, 86, 102
Bleeding, 11
Blindness and claustrophobia, 64
Blindness, temporary, 141
Blindness, temporary, by water in eyes feared, 142
Blindness, temporary, in fever, 164
Blindness, total, 31
Blinds always pulled tight, 135
Blinking eyes with jerking motions, 170
Blinking, 29, 139
Body arched backwards in night terror, 123
Body divided, 32
Body language, 35
Body, 135-177
Body, spirit and vital force, 6
Boenninghausen, 11
Bonding by child with homeopath, 61
Bonding problems and *Stramonium* state, 174
Bonding severed by child, 62

Bonding, difficulties, 60 - 61, 70
Bonding, problems with fetus, 60
Bone breaking, threat of, 73
Bones of statue in dreams, 124
*Borax*, 117
Boring head into pillow in fever, 163
Born alone and dies alone, realization that one is, 106
Born underweight and *Stramonium* state, 174
Bossiness, 43, 144
Bouncing off walls, 90
Bowel movement preceded by abdominal pain, 158
Brain affected by infection, 76
Brain diseases, organic, 135
Brain injuries as etiology in nervous system disorders, 171
Brain trauma and seizures, 138
Brain, fever and dehydration, 159
Brain, new, and old, 19
Brain, speech centers, 146
Breach of consciousness by unconsciousness increases in night terrors, 126
Bread as play lethal weapon, 85
Breakfast, aversion to, 156
Breast, mother scratched, in dentition, 146
Breast feeding aggravates, 156
Breasts obsession with, 160
Breath, shortness of, aggravated by lying, 153
Breathing deeply and relaxation as sign of established contact in night terrors, 128
Breathing laborious, fast and short, 152
Breathing, cessation of, 31
Brittle quality, 110
Bronchitis after remedy, requiring repeat of *Stramonium*, 154
Bronchitis and autism, 108
Bronchitis in infancy, 151
Bronchitis, 52, 150-152, 155, 174
Bronchitis, dry nose, initial heat phase, 146
Brother, hated, 21
Brutality, 81
*Bryonia alba*, 152-153
*Bufo*, 16, 94
Bugs, fear of, 51, 53
Buildings in dreams, 124
Bullies, 63, 72
Bumping head causes temper tantrum in headache, 137

192

Buried alive, 34, 106
Buried alive, delusion of being, 62, 63
Burrowing head in pillow in meningitis, 172
Burrowing in blankets, 30, 132
Bystanders, hit, 85

*Calcarea carbonica* mother's fright creates in newborn *Stramonium* state, 173
*Calcarea carbonica*, 17, 20, 21, 122, 156
*Calcarea phosphorica*, 16, 88, 117
*Calcareas*, 16
Calm, during fever, 52
Camera, held to face, fear of, 52
Canker sores, 147
*Cannabis indica*, 16
Capriciousness, 32, 95, 144, 156
Car accidents as etiology in nervous system disorders, 171
Car crashes, 51
Car seat, 49
Caresses, adverse to in fever, 143
Carnivores, fear of, 53
Carried, better from being, 13
Carried, desires to be, 12
Case interview, observations in, 97
Case of allergic reaction, 165-166
Case of anaphylactic shock from antibiotics, 149
Case of asthma, 153
Case of autism, 107-108
Case of birth trauma, 109
Case of bladder surgery, 177
Case of depression, 102
Case of desire to kill, 21
Case of encephalitis, 172
Case of epilepsy, 167, 168
Case of fever, 164
Case of Halloween witch and hyperactivity, 176-177
Case of headache with nightmares, 51
Case of hyperactivity, 91
Case of hyperactivity with fiendish laughter, 81-84
Case of joy of violence, 85
Case of learning disability, 97
Case of lymphoma, cured by *Stramonium*, xi
Case of meningitis, 171
Case of nightmares, 66
Case of night terrors, 53, 122-124

Case of night terror after vaccination, 152
Case of one month old, temper tantrums, in, 85
Case of punishing (policeman) behavior, 80-81
Case of ritualism, autism and violence, 109-110
Case of seizures, 65, 168-169
Case of seizures after DPT, 176
Case of severe eczema, 165-166
Case of temper tantrum, 79-80
Case of temper tantrums and perseverative behavior, 77-79
Case of vaginal bleeding, 11
Case of violence and family stress, 69, 72
Case management, 89
Case taking, more effective way, xiii
Catalog of tortures, as if leafing through, 139
Cats, 53
Caution, 55, 67
Cemeteries, see graveyards
Central Nervous System, see CNS
Cerebral Palsy, 109, 174
Cervical glands enlarged, in infection, causing neck pain, 163
Cervical glands swollen, 149
Cesarean section, 70
Chafing, red skin, 148
Chained, delusion of being, in night terrors, 129
Chain saw, 49
Chameleon nature of *Stramonium*, 37
*Chamomilla*, 117, 136, 146-147
Chaos as world view, 57
Chaos, 94
Characteristic symptoms, 7
Chasing, 81
Cheese, craves, 156
Chest and bronchi, (right side) ears and nose, (left side) 145
Chest constriction in asthma, 153
Chest, oppression of, like weight on, 152
Chewing in seizure, 168
Child beaten by parent, 177
Child bites toy dog, 82
Child given away, 177
Child responds to frightening situation the same as mother did, 173
Child's face, water thrown at, 64

193

Chills and fevers, 163-164
Chills felt in back and extremities, 163
Choking and swallowing after DPT vaccination, 149
Choking brings *Stramonium* state, 165
Choking family members, 84
Choking, 62, 149, 152
Chorea, 29
Choreic motion of left hand and arm, 169
Christmas mass, 51
Chronic disease and overreaction, 29
Chronic disease, and vital force, 6
Chronic low level fear, 45
*Cina*, 117, 146-147
Circular hand motions in tighter and tighter circles, 169
Cities, weird and scary, in dreams, 124
Citrus aggravated, red skin, 148
Citrus and canker sores, 147
Citrus, craves, 156
Civil disobedience, 49
Civilizing passions, 34
Clarity, loss of, 57
Clarity, strived for, 112
Claustrophobia, 59, 62 -63
Claustrophobic effect of darkness, 58
Clawing, 54, 73, 75
Cleanliness, 111, 112
Clenching in seizure, 168
Climbing curtains in night terror, 123
Climbing, 82
Clinging, 25, 28, 29, 33, 45, 46, 61, 67, 70, 117, 144, 149, 153, 166
Clingy in earache and fever, 143
Close, Stewart, 4
Closed behavior, 100
Closes one eye then both, 169
Closet, hiding in, 63, 71
Closets, fear of, 59, 62, 65
Closing off segment, 25, 27, 30-33, 60, 63, 85, 103, 112
Closing off, as protection, 27
Clothes obsessions, 109, 111
Clothes, dirty, 94
Clothes, displaying violent words and images, 85
Clothes, rips, 86
Clowning, 52, 95
Clues from simply observing child, 81

CNS dysfunction in mother sends infant to *Stramonium* state, 173
Coat hangers as guns, 87
Cobra, spitting, fear of, 55
Coffin, delusion of being in, 154
Coition at young age, 160
Cold air aggravates asthma, 153
Cold ameliorates headache, 137
Cold tar, used in impetigo, 165
Coldness, 31
Colds ameliorates yet aggression increases, 87
Colds cease after remedy given, 145
Colds repeated in infancy, 174
Colic, 56, 112
Color black, of anything, named to ameliorate fear, 141
Colors, dark, fear of, 59
Colors, loved, 111
Coma, in and out of for weeks in encephalitis, 172
Comfort foods, 12, 157
Comfort seeking, 10, 12, 13, 32, 33, 44, 76, 80
Commands must be repeated by parent, 145
Commands refused, 66
Communicate, desire to, 30, 33
Communication difficulties, 99
Communication improved, 105
Communication skills lost, 113
Company, aversion, yet dreads being alone, 143
Company, desires, yet treats them outrageously, 143
Comparison of *Stramonium* with *Lycopodium* and *Medorrhinum*, 43
Complaining, 66
Complications of labor and birth and *Stramonium* state, 174
Comprehension, slowness in, 98
Compulsive behavior, 46
Compulsive wiping after bowel movement, 158
Computer games, limiting, 68
Concentration span poor, 96, 97
Conception, moment of, 6
Concepts, difficulty grasping, 96
Condition of child; parent and doctor putting themselves in place, 145
Confidence lacking, xi
Confidence after remedy, 67

194

Confined spaces preferred, 63
Confined spaces, as birth canal, 56
Confined, fear of being, 66
Confining activities, as hugging, causing fear, 62
Confrontation, fear of, 86
Confusion about identity segment, see also Dual states
Confusion and mania, 32
Confusion brings on fear causing violence, 75
Confusion of dream and reality, 120
Confusion of reality, 27, 31
Confusion of self and reality, 76
Confusion, 28, 32, 57, 77, 78, 98, 118
Congestive headaches, 136
Conjunctivitis and photophobia, 141
Conjunctivitis, 142
Connecting to others, 44
Conscientious over trifles, 112
Conscious and unconscious world, stuck between, 75
Conscious control relinquished, 115
Conscious during seizures, 167
Conscious enjoyment of violence, 76, 80-84, 85, 92, 94
Conscious mind, 35
Conscious mind, loss of control over, 113
Conscious side blinded by water, 64
Conscious side frightened and overcontrolled, 168
Conscious violence, unconscious violence, and state between, 77
Conscious world, 75
Consciousness and unconsciousness, struggle between, in night terror, 122
Consciousness vs. unconsciousness, 34 see also Dual nature, 34
Consequences and punishment out of the question, 73
Consequences of treating wrong layer, 23
Consistency, lack of, 95
Consolation, desires 12, 13
Consolation, importance of, in night terrors, 120
Constipation and diarrhea alternating, xi
Constipation, 21
Constitutional needs, 18
Constitutional states, 21, 126
Constriction of throat, 149

Contemplation, profound, appears to be in, 97
Contractions, 12
Contradiction and violence to self, 86
Contradictions within remedy, 66-67
Contradictory fears, 56
Contradictory symptoms, 39
Contrary behavior, 83
Control of others, 109
Control strategy at bedtime, 118
Control, loss of eye motions, 140
Control, see over-control, 125
Controlling others with violence, 72
Controlling side, 117
Convergent strabismus, 140
Conversations in sleep, 132
Convulsion begins at extremities and moves upwards, 168
Convulsions alternating with excitement, 72
Convulsions from glittering objects, 30
Convulsions with consciousness, 34, 167-168
Convulsions, rage during, 74
Cope, inability to, 78
Cornered, feeling of being, 58
Cortex and the new brain, 34
Cortex, overriding hypothalamus, in night terrors, 130
Cosmology of remedies, 24
Cough causing vomiting, 144
Cough, 38 52, 53, 155
Cough, incessant during sleep, 151
Cough, leading to vomiting, 153
Cough, rattling, 152
Coughing, interminable, 151
Coughs, ameliorated yet aggression increases, 87
Coughs, spasmodic and teasing, 152
Counseling, 71, 101
Courage, lack of, 43
Crabby, 72
Cramping, 12, 30
Crawling on floor during sleep, 132
Crimes, heinous, 35
Criteria, of new homeopathic model, 4
Cross eyed, 140
Cross-wise symptoms, left upper, right lower, 175
Croup, 151
Croup, recurring and asthma, 153
Crowded places, acting out in, 47

Crowds, fear of, 13, 48
Cruel humor, 95
Cruelty, 73, 81
Crushed, delusion of being, in night terrors, 129
Crying of parent in response to night terror, 123
Crying, 45, 56, 66, 67, 79, 102, 110
Cuddly, 66
Cunning demeanor, 82
Cursing in Tourette's syndrome, 170
Cut throat, threatens to, 71
Cuts self with razor, 86, 103
Cutting self premenstrually, 161
Cycle of abuse and punishment, 120
Cycle of remedy and nuances, 39
Cycle of ritual to fear and violence, 109
Cycle of *Stramonium* remedies, 3-14, 27-35, 32-35, 38, 60, 74, 75, 121
Cycle, flow of, 13
Cycles reinforced, 9
Cycles, simplified or contracted, 35

Dairy aggravates, skin red, 148
Dairy, craved, except in infants, 156
Dancing, 73
Danger lurking, 44
Danger, as if in, between sleep and waking, 122
Dante, 44
Dark room ameliorates headache, 137
Dark side, 47, 50
Dark, 44, 53, 54, 57, 60-61, 65, 66, 67, 71, 96, 112, 116, 119, 149, 153, 154
Darkness vs. light, 32
Darkness, desire for, 60
Darkness, fear of, as fear of injury, 57
Darkness, world of, 34
Daydreaming, 93
Dead feeling, 27
Dead people rising, 51-52
Dead segment of child, 29
Dead, as if, 137, 139
Dead, that one side of him is, 32
Dead, wishes he were, 86
Deafness, temporary, 117
Death and deadness, 31
Death segment, 140, see Shut down

Death wish and life wish, precarious balance of, 32
Death, fear of, 25, 28, 30, 33, 44, 50, 51, 53, 66
Decapitating toy dog, 82
Deep sleep, waking from and night terrors, 121
Defeated by life, 95
Defecate, inability to, 31
Defense mechanism and flaw in, 29
Defensive violence, 46
Defiling dead bodies, 135
Dehydration, 158
Delirium, fever, delusions in, 163
Delirium and facial skin infections, 148
Delirium in fever, 76
Delirium in infections, 149
Delirium, 43, 60, 144, 153, 159
Delirium, holding genitals, in meningitis, 172
Delusions of half buried, half dead, half alive, 34
Delusions, xi, 37, 53, 100
Demanding, 29
Demonic behavior, 19, 116, 175
Demonic retribution, fear of, 50
Demonic side craves lemons, 157
Demons, talks to, 100
Denial, 79
Dentition, 146
Dentition, slow, 21
Depression and suicidal impulse alternates with anger, 103
Depression, 31, 45, 47, 102-103
Deserted, delusion of being, 60
Desire, singular, for only one thing, 92
Desires thwarted, 91, 92, 93
Desires to kill himself, 102
Desperation, 32, 33
Destructive behavior, 83, 84, 91
Detachment, 75
Developmental delays, 112, 169
Devil, seeing, since encephalitis, 172
Devils in *Hyoscyamus* and *Stramonium*, 50
Devils, 31, 50, 65, 87, 125, 129, 153
Diabolic laughter, 82
Diaper changing, aversion to, 158
Diaper changing in night terrors, 129
Diaphragm strained in respiratory infection causes back pain, 162

196

Diaphragm, involuntary jerking motion of, 170
Diarrhea in dentition, 146
Diarrhea, 29, 35, 158
Diarrhea, sour and offensive, 158
Diary, craves, 156
Die soon, believes he will, 172
Die, as if he will, in night terror, 124
Differential diagnosis of case and physical symptoms, 175
Differentiating acceptable behaviors, 106
Digestive tract, sensitive to acidic foods, 147
Direction of cure, 17, 21
Disappears within himself, 108
Discharges, excessive, 29
Discoloration, red, ear, 143
Disease, cyclical nature of, 10, 67
Dislike of child by father, 174
Disobedience, 93-94
Disruptive behavior, 93
Distant feeling of father to child, 174
Distracted easily, 97
Divided body, 32
Divine comedy, the, 44
Divorce, 69, 116, 154
Dizziness and encephalitis, 172
Do not go gentle into that good night, by Dylan Thomas, 69
Doctor, as torturer, 49
Dogs imagined as big carnivores, 53
Dogs, 52, 65, 80, 83, 109, 126, 128
Dolls, 83
Domineering, 73
Doors closed, fear of, 62
Door, locking, 13, 59
Doorway to the unconscious, 19
Double vision, 140
Dowsing, fear of, 64
DPT and strabismus, 140
DPT vaccine and hypoglycemia, 156
DPT vaccine and loss of mental ability, 176
DPT vaccine and swallowing difficulties, 149
DPT vaccine, and *Stramonium* state, 150
Drama of vital force, 6-7
Dramatic affect of night terrors on parents, 124
Dramatic layer, 24
Draw, desire to, 87
Draw, inability to, 98

Dreams of abuse and violence, 161
Dreams of violence, 103
Dreams, terrifying, fear of, 116
Drinking habits, 110
Drinks, cold, aggravates asthma, 153
Drinks, cold, thirst for, 163
*Drosera*, 151-152
Drug interactions and asthma treatment, 155
Drug reaction and hives, 165
Dry cough, 150
Drying, importance of, bed wetting *Stramonium* child, 129
Dual state of consciousness, 31-32
Duality and sleep behavior, 122
Duality in sexual behavior, 162
Duality in *Stramonium* shown in food aversions and cravings, 155-157
Duality of food, desires and aversions, 156-157
Duality of remedy in pale or red facial color, 147
Dullness and anesthesia, 96
Dullness becomes violence, 20
Dullness, 20, 89, 96
Dullness, as reaction to fear, 98
Dumb look, 71
Dumb since Halloween, 107
Dying alone, 51, 106
Dying, obsession with, 66
Dynamic aspect of remedy, 7
Dyslexic, 96, 97

Ear infection and pain, 142-145
Ear infection poorly treated and meningitis, 171
Ear infection, 52, 56, 174
Earache, 13, 112, 155
Earache, aggravated by heat, 143
Earache, ameliorated, warmth and bundling, 143
Earaches, acute, 142-143
Earaches, sudden onset, 143
Ears, 142-145
Ears, red, 84
Ears, sensitive to noise in meningitis, 171
Eaten by a monster, about to be, 177
Eating ceased for two weeks after DPT, 176
Eating habits, 110
Echolalia in Tourette's syndrome, 170

Eczema followed by asthma at one year, 174
Eczema within first two months, 174
Eczema, 51, 86, 164-166, 177
EEG changes, 113
EEG findings in seizures, 167
Effect of remedy in night terror, 130
Eggs, aversion to, 156
Electric storm enjoyed, 175
Element, see segment
Elevators, fear of, 62
Eliot, T.S., 7, 105
Elusive quality, 108
Embarrassment, 48, 85
Emergency room, 149, 153, 172
Emergency room, trip to, as etiology, 160
Emotional abuse, 61
Emotional changes following allopathic treatment of rashes, 164
Emotional changes following antipathic treatment of eczema, 164
Emotional needs, goal overshot, 30
Emotional symptoms, 23
Emotional turmoil and red face, 147
Emotional violence, 69
Emotions, whirlpool of, 101
Encephalitis in mother, history of, 173
Encephalitis, 172
Enclosed, being, fear of, 62
Energy conserving, 33
Energy high all day, 175
Energy loss, 31
Enlightenment, spiritual, 60
Environmental factors, 6
Epidemic of children needing *Stramonium*, 38
Epilepsy, 35, 106
Epilepsy, with or without abnormal EEG, 167
Epileptic and newborns, 11
Episodic depression, 95
Episodic violence, 92
Erysipelas, 148
Escape and fear, 46
Escape attempts in night terror, 122
Escape, desire to, 28, 45, 59, 76, 82, 144
Escaped prisoner, like a, 44
Etiology for *Stramonium* in mother 173
Etiology of nervous system disorders, 171
Euphrasia, 142
Event of night terror forgotten in morning, 122
Events, processing, inability to, 79

Evil-doers, vulnerability to, 47
Evil entity, 53, 126
Evil pursued by, dreams of, 161
Evil, fear of, 44, 50
Evil, look of, expressed in eyes, 139
Exaggeration of symptoms in suppressed case, 88
Excitability of nervous system, 89
Excitement alternating with convulsions, 72
Exhaustion and closing off, 30-31
Exhaustion, 13, 33, 101
Exhibitionism, 160
Expectations, harsh self, 55
Expectoration, thick, white, turns yellow-green, bloody in pneumonia, 153
Explosion of destructive energy, 75
Expression of eyes, 139
Extremities stiff in seizures, 168
Extremities uncovered, cold to touch, 163
Extremities, 162-163
Extremities, temperature, during ear infection with fever, 143
Extroverted, 100
Eye contact missing, 110
Eye control, loss in seizures and fevers, 140
Eye infection, 142
Eye problems, 140
Eye rolling, 140
Eyelids moving in side to side direction, 140
Eyelids, twitching and blinking, 139
Eyes as extension of brain, 64
Eyes glaring look, 172
Eyes glazed with fear in fever, 164
Eyes opened and closed in night terror, 123
Eyes rolled up in encephalitis, 172
Eyes, 139-142
Eyes, glazed, 108
Eyes, gritty, sandy sensation, 142
Eyes, sensitive to light, in meningitis, 171
Eyes, terror filled in night terror, 123
Eyes, water in, causes paralyzes, 64

Face red in seizures, 168
Face scratched terribly at night in impetigo, 165
Face, 147-148
Face, red, 79, 84, 163
Face, scratching own, 85
Faces, delusion of, 153

Faces, diabolical, delusion of, 53
Faces, fear of, 53
Faces, making, 91
Faces, painted, 52, 70
Facial color, 147-148
Facial expression intense in Tourette's syndrome, 170
Facial skin infections and delirium, 148
Facial tics in Tourette's syndrome, 170
Facial tics, 148
Failure, 95, 97
Falling gait, 170
Falling out of chair, 77
Falling, 54, 79
Falls off bed in night terror, 124
Family bed, pro and cons, 118, 119
Family pictures draws, 87
Fantasies of killing or being killed, 102
Fantasy of family troubles to be resolved by own suicide, 103
Far away look, 97, 172
Farsighted from early age, 140
Fastidiousness and ritual behavior, 111
Fastidiousness, 153
Fate, abandoned to, 118
Father abuses mother, child fearful since, 177
Father's history of emotional outbursts, 174
Father, whom he hated, 86
Fear in night terrors, 130
Fear on face at start of seizure, 168
Fear with violence, 43
Fear, 23, 32, 43-68, 90, 94, 99, 105, 122, 159, 169, 174
Fear, responses to, 45
Fear, unacknowledged, after sexual abuse, 162
Fear/clinging segment, see also Vulnerability, Death, and Injury.
Feared, better than being loved, 109
Fearful in meningitis, 138
Fearlessness, 67
Fears, flooded with, 106
Fears, following antipathic treatment of eczema, 164
Fears, named reassuringly during night terrors, 128
Febrile seizures, 163
Febrile seizures, effect of remedies, 167
Feeling evoked by *Stramonium* presence, 35

Feelings hurt, 72, 85
Feelings named in night terror transforming effect of, 130
Feet cool in headache with hot head, 137
Ferber Richard, 116, 121, 125
Fetal position, retreat to, 61
Fetus experiences mother's reaction to fright, 173
Fetus, experiences fright of movie, 107
Fever and photophobia, 60, 141
Fever of 104 degrees, 152
Fever spike, 70
Fever, 52, 53, 76, 140, 163-164
Fever, eyes open in, 140
Fever, high with earache, 143
Fever, in menses, flow stops and starts, offensive and dark, 161
Fevers affecting brain during pregnancy, 173
Fevers and eye rolling, 140
Fevers and jerking head off pillow, 170
Fevers and red face, 147
Fevers as etiology in nervous system disorders, 171
Fiendish grin, 85
Fiendish laughter, 82
Fight or flight in seizures, 168
Fight or flight syndrome, 46, 90
Film violence, 84
Fingers clenched in seizure, 168
Fingers pressed into head in headaches, 136
Fingers, keeping separated, 112
Fingers, obsessed with clean, 111
Fist fights, 72, 85
Fit, tumultuous, 102
Fits of unconsciousness and meningitis, 171
Five segments of *Stramonium* cycle, 28-32
Flailing, 76
Fleeing strangers, 47
Flow of symptoms, 28
Flower beds as similar to symptom groups, 10
Flu and autism, 108
Fluid action of chronic diseases, 9
Fluid in ear, 145
Fluidity as opposed to rigid ritualistic behavior, 64
Focal seizures, 168
Focus, 94
Follow-up of case, not waiting for, 87-88

Follow-up, cases lost in, 38
Food allergies and eczema, 165
Food allergy, 151
Food as comforters, 12
Food cravings and aversions, 7
Food obsessions, 109
Foods, mixed, dislike of, 110
Forehead wrinkled, 148
Forehead, as locus of headache, 136
Forehead, wrinkled, in meningitis, 171
Foreskin infection, 160
Forsaken feeling in abuse, 61
Forsaken, feeling of being, 60, 61, 99, 100, 102
Fountains, fear of, 63
*Four Quartets*, of T.S. Eliot, 7, 105
Fresh air ameliorates headache, 137
Friends, cannot make, 99, 135
Fright and stammering, 146
Fright as etiology, 176
Fright preceding illness, 52
Fright, 75
Fright, requiring *Tuberculinum* then *Stramonium*, 22
Frights as etiology in seizures, 171
Frights during day expressed as fears of bedtime, 120
Frogs, fear of, 54
Frozen by terror, 54
Fruit, 12
Fruits, craves, 156
Frustration in case taking, 5
Frustration of parents in night terrors, 124
Frustration, 77, 78, 85, 102, 110, 113
Full autism, 112-114
Fundamental segments of remedy picture, see Segments, fundamental
Funny feeling in head as aura before seizures, 138
Furniture destroyed in seizure, 76
Furniture possesses ghosts, 51
Furniture, hiding behind, 63
Furniture, rearranging, 111
Fury, 73, 74
Future disease, potential for, 17
Future materia medicas, 14
Future predicted, 46

Gags and tricks, as etiology, 62
Gait, funny or odd appearance of, 170
Games, solitary, 107
Gender and remedy description, xiv
Gender mistakes in speech, 96
Genetics factors, 6
Genitals touched too forcefully, 160
Genitals, holding, 160
Genitals, own, grabs, 83
Genitals, punches mother in, 84
Gentler after remedy, 87
Germs, 3, 66
Gestures by child in night terrors indicating parent contact established, 128
Gestures, see Hands
Ghegas, Vassilis, M.D., poetic comment on vitiligo, 165
Ghostly delusions in fever, 144
Ghosts in dreams, 121
Ghosts, 31, 50, 51, 53, 54, 57, 65, 66, 87, 125
Giggling, demonic, 141
Gilles de la Tourette, see Tourette's syndrome
Girls, 161-162
Glans, red and swollen, 160
Glare of sun, aversion to, 175
Glass broken, fear of, 61
Glass of water, fear of in meningitis, 171
Glee, 83
Glittering objects and convulsions, 30
Gloating laughter, 81
Goodman, Benny, 5
Grabbing, 83
Graceful motions, as if swimming, 169
Graphic descriptions of terror, violence, 38
Grave, in, delusion of being, 62, 63
Graveyards, 51
Gray zone of case analysis, 5
Grid, remedies located on, 18
Grid, upper and lower phase four, 20
Grief from reaction of loved ones, 101
Grief, from, tears at face and rips eyes out, 166
Grieving, 71
Grimacing, 89, 148
Grinning, 77
Growling, 81
Guarded and depressed, 47
Guilt allayed by discussion of stress and conflicts helping night terrors, 125
Guilt, 70, 117
Guns, obsession with, 78, 110
Guttural laughter and tones, 54, 83, 169

200

Hahnemann, Samuel, 3, 8, 21, 181-186
Hair washing in the morning, to curtail night terrors, 127
Hair washing, fear of, 63, 126
Hair, own, tears out, 86
Hairy, delusions in fever, 144
Half alive, dream of being, 124
Half dead side shuns light, 142
Halloween, 107
Hallucinatory deliriums in fever, 144
Hallucinogenic, effects of, 39
Hallways, dark, fear of, 59
Hand in pocket, holding genitals, 160
Hand, as if moving by itself, 169
Hands and wrists appear like praying mantis, 169
Hands cool in headache with hot head, 137
Hands perform involuntary actions, 169
Hands severed, 49
Hands, involuntary motions of, 89
Haphazard symptomology, 4
Harmed or hurt, dreams of being, 121
Harshness by parents in child's closed off state, 101
Hate for those who contradict them, 73
Hatred of self, 102
Hatred, 20, 70
Haughtiness, 81
Head bored into pillow in fever, 163
Head bruised, 174
Head drawn back and to one side in seizures, 138
Head hot in headache, yet extremities cool, 137
Head injuries, 135, 136
Head jerked backwards in encephalitis, 172
Head jerks side to side in seizure 168
Head raising off pillow in meningitis, 172
Head submerged in water, 65
Head tilted in seizures, 168
Head, 138
Head, banging on floor, 85
Head, drawn back and to one side in sleep, 132
Head, rolling side to side, 107
Head, wet, fear of, 63
Headache from reflected sunlight, 141
Headache in pneumonia, 152
Headache pain drives child mad, 136

Headache, pain, difficult for child to describe, 136
Headaches in fevers, 163
Headaches, 136-137, 175
Healing, emotional realm and infections developing, 155
Health improved yet more violent, 87
Hearing and ear infections, 145
Hearing disability and autism, 112
Heart chewed by wolf in night terror, 122
Heat aggravates, 175
Heat of sun, aversion to, 175
Heights, fright of, 56
Held, desire to be, 46, 52
Hell, a living, and seeking spiritual light, 60
Hell, as if in, 106, 137
*Helleborus,* 16, 20, 138, 172
Hellish environment, enjoyable, 169
Hering's Law, 17, 21
Hering's Law, in larger scale, of remedy picture, 18
Hernia, 96
Hiccoughs cause back pain, 162
Hideous side of unconscious, 43
Hiding, 67, 106
Hierarchy of remedies and symptoms, 15-24
High fever and vaccines, 176
Hitting himself in Tourette's syndrome, 170
Hitting in meningitis, 171
Hitting self, 79
Hitting, 30, 47, 48, 54, 66, 71, 74, 75, 78, 79, 80, 149
Hives and violence, 165
Hoarseness, 149, 152
Holding on, 12
Home, desire to go, even when at, 153
Homeopathic suppression of eczema and new mental/emotional symptoms, 164-165
Homeopathic, old masters, 37
Horror books, 38
Horror movies, relish and fear of, 39
Horror, 44
Hospital stay as etiology 177
Hospital, 53
Hostile environments, 63
Hot blooded, 142
Hugging and seizures, 167
Hugging in night terrors, conditions for efficacy of, 129

Hugging, 83, 109
Humor, cruel, 95
Humorous behavior, 91
Hurling objects, 85
Hurt, fear of being, 27
Hurting siblings, 80
Hydrocephalus, 135, 136
*Hyoscyamus* and *Stramonium*, similarity and change to, 20
*Hyoscyamus*, 16,17, 18, 20, 81, 84, 92, 94, 96, 113, 149, 159, 160, 162, 169, 170,172
Hyperfocusing, 92-93, 94
Hyper qualities changed by repatterning visual skills, 140
Hypervigilance, 30, 55, 99
Hyperactivity and attention difficulties, 89
Hyperactivity, 11, 15, 84, 86, 96, 98, 108, 113, 142, 150, 158, 177
Hypersensitivity to pain, 137, 176
Hypoglycemia, 156
Hypothalamus and cortex, raging struggle between, 131
Hypothalamus and night terrors, 130
Hypothalamus and the old brain, 34
Hypothalamus, 96
Hysteria from being yelled at, 80
Hysteria, 56, 79

I.Q., 96, 113
Ice Cream, 12
Ice, craves, 156
Identity of self and others confused, 78
Images of being alone, 67
Images of death, 67
Images of horror, 106
Images of violence, 103
Imaginary things and people doing horrible things in fever or delirium, 163
Imaginary threat, 77
Imagination and vulnerability, 49
Imagination, 52, 57, 111
Imagined hurt, 30
Immobility, feeling of, in dark, 58
Impetigo, 149, 165
Important, need to feel, 81
Impressionable nature, 100
Imprisoned, delusion of being, in night terrors, 129
Impulse control improved after remedies, 86

Impulse control in healing process, 131
Impulse control, poor, 89, 92, 94,
Impulse control developing, 117
Impulsive, 15, 74, 81, 84, 89, 98
Inattentive behavior, 93
Incoherent answers, 97
Incommunicative, 100
Inconsolable in headache, 136
Incubator as isolation etiology, 60
Indecision, 32
Indestructibility, sense of, 67
Infant, eye contact lacking, 110
Infection and autism, 108
Infections and CNS and pregnant mother, 173
Infections and jerking head off pillow, 170
Infections as etiology in nervous system disorders, 171
Infections in meningitis, 171
Infections, 15, 54
Infections, respiratory tract, 150
Inferiority complex and mildness, 103
Inflammation in fever, 76
Inflammation of brain, 138
Inflammation of ear, 143
Inflammations, 112
Infolding of psyche, 113
Information, inadequacy of, 15
Ingratitude for previous physically curative remedies in sexual abuse, 162
Inhibitions, loss of, 101
Injury, delusions of, in night terror, 122
Injury to head, 135-136
Injury, delusion, that is about to receive, 145
Injury, fear of, 25, 28, 49, 99, 145
Inner world of his own, 91, 100, 113
Inner world reflected in outer chaos, 94
Inner world vs. control of outer world, 46
Inner world, intrusions into, violent reaction to, 72-74
Inner world, retreat into, 61-62
Innocence denied, 44
Innocent self and horrid dreams, 117
Insanity, 15, 37
Insects, 65
Insecurity in case taking, 5
Insecurity, 43, 48, 145
Insecurity, child's sense of, heightened by seeing violence, 119
Insults, 73

Intelligence above average, yet dumb look, 71
Intensity levels of pathology, 16
Intensity of symptoms compared, 17
Intensity of symptoms, 17, 21, 38
Intention not necessary in violent behavior, 69
Intentional violence, 84
Intermingling of conscious and unconscious, 34, 35
Intertwining of nosode and underlying remedy, 19
Interventions in night terror positive and negative, 125-131
Interview observations, 94
Introversion from extroverted state, 99
Introversion in seizures, 168
Introversion, 45, 47, 74, 99-103, 101, 158
Intrusions, 49
Invasion of her body, dreams terrible, of, 161
Involuntary actions, 169
Involuntary motion, hand circles in front of face, 169
Inwardness, 43
Irrational behavior, 156
Irrational from headache pain, 136
Irritability, 43, 69, 74, 153
Isolation, 62, 71, 86, 100, 105, 106, 107, 118, 125, 174, 177
Isolation, sense of, accentuated by darkness, 58
Itchy, red eyes, 142

Jabbing with pen, 85
Jacksonian march in convulsions, 168
James, William, 40
Jarring aggravates headache, 137
Jaw motion in seizure, 168
Jaws moving back and forth in meningitis, 171
Jealousy, 20
Jealousy, *Hyoscyamus* and *Pulsatilla* compared, 17
Jerking head off pillow, 138, 170
Jerking in sleep, 132
Jerking motions, 170-171
Job interview, 125
Joke, gruesome, known only to himself, 169
Joker, the, 95-96
Jokes, practical, hurtful, 95

Joking and vertigo, 138-139
Joking, 90
Joking, sexual, 96
Joy in case taking, 5
Joy in terror and violence, 76, 80-85, 92, 94
Juices, craves, 156
Jumping, 73
Jung, Carl, 19, 47, 64, 120
Justice meted out by child, 80

Keynote head symptom, 138
Keynotes to *Stramonium*, 34
Keynotes, not commonly seen in *Stramonium*, 138
Keynotes, phase one, remedy, 23
Keynotes, literal interpretation, 10
Keynotes, xiii
Kicking, 71, 73, 74, 75, 77, 78, 79, 84, 92, 102, 172
Kicks in night terror, 123
Kidney disease and pregnant mother, brain affected by, 173
Kidney infections in pregnancy, 70
Kill, threatens to, 71
Killed, feeling of being, in night terror, 122
Killing off parts of self, 33
Killing or being killed, fantasies of, 102
Killing, attempts at, 113
Kill self, desire to, in headache pain, 136
Kinesthetic sense of remedy, xiv
Kissed, adverse to being, in fever, 143
Kisses father after remedy, 86
Kissing in night terrors, conditions for efficacy of, 129
Knee to chest, 132
Knives and razors to cut self, premenstrually, 161
Knives, evokes stabbing, 49
Knives, obsession with, 110
Knowledge pool, developing a, 7

Labor complications and difficult bonding, 60
Labor, difficult, of several days, and *Stramonium* state, 174
Lachesis, 82, 96, 113, 136, 149
Ladders, fright on, 56
Lake, fear of, 127
Landau-Kleffner syndrome, 106, 112-114

Language, invents, 95, 96
Laryngitis, 150
Laughing and staring through doctor, 169
Laughing, 148
Laughter and hyperactivity, 81-84
Laughter, diabolic, 19, 82
Laughter, doubling over with, 95
Laughter, gloating, 81-84
Laughter, guttural, 83
Laughter, strange, 91
Lawton, Jeenet, 99
Layer and sexual abuse, 161
Layer, consequences of treating wrong, 23
Layers, 21, 23, 101
Layers, treating, respective, 87
Learning capacity, experiential, 67
Learning difficult since encephalitis, 172
Learning impairments, 65, 97
Left eye involuntarily closed, right eye staring, 141
Left hand, common site of rashes, 164
Left side predominates in seizures, 167
Left side symptoms of eyes, ears and nose, 175
Left sided head injuries, 135
Legs eaten in night terror, 122
Legs, 111
Lemons, craves, 156
Lethargy in encephalitis, 172
Lethe, 115
Life vs. death, 35
Life wish and death wish, precarious balance of, 32
Lifeline through child, in night terrors, 130
Light aggravates headache, 137
Light and water, 141-142
Light during sleep, turned off by parents, 119
Light forces, 116
Light in bedroom for night terrors, 127
Light perceived as fire, 122
Light vs. darkness, 32
Light, desire for, 59
Light, fear of, 60
Light, sensitivity to, 12, 30
Light, world of, 34
Lightning storms, fear of or delight in, 49, 66
Lights and cessation of night terror, 123
Lights, screaming for, even when lights are on, 141

Lights, sudden, 49
Limb, numbness of, 31
Limbic system and the old brain, 34
Limbic system, 96, 144
Limiting, potential fear situations, 67-68
Linguistic ability, average or above, 114
Lions, 53, 66
Lips moving back and forth in meningitis, 171
Lips, red, 149
Listlessness in fever, 152
Listlessness, 89
Literature and kinesthetics of remedy, xiv
Live, desire to, 30, 33, 138
Live, desire to, and food cravings, 157
Live, desire to, mutilated, 44
Live, desire to, overshot, 31-32
Live, not wishing to, 29-30
Locked in closet, as *Stramonium* etiology, 59
Locking doors, 67
Logical pattern of symptoms, 8
Logical totality of symptoms, 4
Loneliness, 70
Loose stools, 158, 174
Loquacity, 95-96
Love life, disappointments in, xi
Love, anguished in parents, 105
Loved ones, driven away, 29
Loving to father after remedy, 86
Loving words in night terrors, 129
Lower respiratory tract, 150-155
Lucretius, 174
Lulling himself, 98
Lurking entity, 50
*Lycopodium*, 16, 22-23, 88, 109, 117, 148, 154, 160, 163
Lymphoma, xi
*Lyssinum*, 85, 136

Machiavelli, Niccolo, 109
Magnification of fears by darkness, 57
Maliciousness, 86
*Mancinella*, 16
Mania and confusion, 32
Mania remedies, 37
Mania, 37, 60
Manic episode, 59
Manipulation, see Control
Mannequin heads, fear of, 51

Map of hierarchy, 15-25, 34, 37
Mask of action, 47
Masks and seizures, 171
Masks, 50, 52, 107, 144
Masturbation, 94
Masturbation, after abuse, 162
Materia medica of the future, 14
Materia Medica Viva, by George Vithoulkas, xi
Materia medica, xi, 12, 15, 138, 148, 163
Materia medica, expanding on, 27
Materia medicas, old people and the mentally and emotionally challenged, xiii
Matrix language for classical homeopaths, 7
Maze, fear of, 62
Meanness, calculated, 46
Measles, 52
Meat, dislikes, xi
Meats, smoked and fatty, craves, 156
Meats, tough, aversion to, 156
Media culture society, 38
Media, inflammation of, 143
Medical advice on night terrors, evaluated, 129
Medical literature, advice on night terrors, 125
Meditation in water, 64
*Medorrhinum*, 16, 17, 18, 40, 87, 103, 117, 132, 142, 156-157, 158, 163, 175
*Medorrhinum*, shared symptoms with *Stramonium* and *Baryta carbonica*, 20
Melville, Herman, 64, 117
Memories of abuse repressed, 161
Memorizing vs. understanding, 8
Meningitis as etiology in nervous system disorders, 171
Meningitis, 70, 76, 135, 136, 138, 144, 171-172
Meningitis, progression of: chills, fever, vomiting, headache, convulsions, 171
Menses, painful, extending to groin and thighs, 161
Mental ability lost after vaccination, 176
Mental rigidity, 112
Mental state, 7
Mental symptoms, xiii
Merry go round: infection, antibiotic, infection, antibiotic, 152
Mesmerized, 54
Message of vital force, 6
Messages mixed, to nervous system, 30

Metaphor of water, 64
Metaphysical obsessions, 66
Meticulousness, 74
Miasms and food cravings, 157
Miasms, 3
Miasms and polychrests bridged, 14
Mildness, xi
Milk aggravates asthma, 176
Milk, aversion to, 156
Milk, especially cold, craves, 156
Mime of violence, 44
Mimicking actions, of others, 78-79
Mimicry of violence as thrill, 81
Mind rubrics, 60
Mind, focusing difficulties, 93
Miracles in treating full autism, 114
Mirror of inner turmoil, 44
Mirror of stresses in nightmares, 120
Mirror symptoms of distressed vital force, 6
Misbehaving if not well rested, 176
Miscarriage, threatened, from face washing, 11
Mischievous, 52, 82
Miserable feeling, 95
Mistrust, 14
Misunderstandings and lashing out, 92
Misunderstood, 33, 110
Mixed up foods, aversion to, 156
MMR vaccine and behavioral problems, 148
Moaning in sleep and night terrors, 123, 132
Moaning, 48, 54
Moby Dick, 64
Models, new, to fit observations and insights into homeopathic phenomena, 4-6, 22
Monomania, 93
Monsters and seizures, 167
Monsters as non-issue after remedy in night terrors, 130
Monsters, 50, 57, 67, 83, 87, 116, 117, 130
Monsters, dream of, 66, 121; 161
Mood swings, 95
Morning irritability, 74
Mother disappearing around corner causing panic, 126
Mother experiences fetus' reaction to her fright, 173
Mother's soothing words, to no avail, 117
Mother, father, pregnancy and newborn, 173-174

Mother, petrified on a windy sea, 111
Motion, sudden, 49
Motions, involuntary, 169
Motions, uncontrolled, in Tourette's syndrome, 170
Motor coordination poor, 66, 72
Motor overflow, 77-79, 93, 98
Motorcycle guy in dreams, 124
Motto, of Hahnemann, 3
Mouth, 146-147
Mouth, dry, 163
Move, desire to, 30
Movie images in dreams, 121
Movie theaters, dark, fear of, 59
Movie violence, 119
Movies, 38, 54, 61, 67, 70, 116, 126, 130
Movies, scary, 50, 51
Movies, violent, discouraged to eliminate night terrors, 127
Mr. MacGregor, 68, 81
Mr. Roger's show, fear from, 70
Mumps and pale face, 147
Mumps, behavioral problems after, 148
Murder, attempted, 21
Muscles taught and tense in fever, 164
Muscular origin of abdominal pains, 158
Muscular strain in respiratory illness causes back pain, 162
Musculoskeletal system, 162, 163
Museum, fear of, 65
Myoclonus, 168

Nails driven into eyes, dream of, 66
Nails, bites, 86
Naming night terror transforms feelings, 130
Naming of fears ameliorates, 140
Naming of stress to diminish (Step 2), 126
Naming trigger stimuli of night terrors, (Step 4), 126
Naps, short, in afternoon enabling late nights, 175-176
Narrow places, fear of, 62
Nasal discharge when eating and in cold air, 146
*Natrum muriaticum*, 55, 100, 101, 103, 156
*Natrums*, 16
Natural occurrences vs. evil-doers, 47
Nature pictures, draws, 87
Nausea in the morning, 156

Nearsighted from early age, 140
Neat, xi
Neck drawn sideways in seizure, 168
Neglect, 99
Negotiating with parents, 93
Nervous breakdown in father's history, 174
Nervous system and eyes, 139-140
Nervous system disorders, etiology of, 171
Nervous system symptoms categorized, 166
Nervous system, 29, 30, 33, 148
Nervous system, symptoms of, 138
Neuralgic ear pain, ameliorated by warmth, 143
Neurodermatitis and hives, 165
Neurologic explosions, 75-76
Neurologic response, quick, 69
Neurologic signs, 89
Neurological disorders, 15, 106, 132
Neurological symptoms, xi
Neutral nature of unconscious, 19
New brain and cortex, 34
Newborn with low pulse and little body tone, 174
Newton, Sir Issac, 3
Night terror, contents extrapolated from nightmares, 122
Night terrors discussed openly with older children, 125
Night terrors in pneumonia, 153
Night terrors resembling and in seizures, 167-168
Night terrors temporarily increased as violence decreases after remedy, 131
Night terrors triggered by noise or touch, 121
Night terrors, 32, 34, 53, 54, 59, 63, 70, 71, 75, 80, 113, 114, 116, 120-130, 120, 121, 152, 172, 175
Night terrors, four step method to dispel, 126-131
Night terrors, intensity of, 122
Night terrors, not outgrown, 125-126
Night terrors, preceded by abdominal pains before bedtime, 158
Night terrors, triggers named, 126
Night, 154
Night, aggravation of stuffed nose, 146
Night, primeval, cosmic, 120
Nightmare and REM sleep, 120
Nightmare themes, 121, 124

206

Nightmares, 51, 54, 62, 66, 116, 120-131, see also Dreams
Nightmarish view of life, 49
Nighttime aggravation with earache, 143
Nipples twisted, 80
Noise and earache, 143
Noise triggering night terrors, 121
Noise, 12, 30, 49, 65, 73, 80, 93, 109
Non communication, 31
Non-interference with night terrors, 125
Nose bleeding, 11
Nose stopped up, 31
Nose, 145-146
Nose, running, dries up, 146
Nosebleeds at night, 146
Nosodes and *Hyoscyamus*, 20
Nosodes and layers: *Sulphur, Medorrhinum, Calcarea, Tuberculinum* compared, 19
Nosodes in phase two, 19
Nosodes, 37, 38, 157
Novels, horror, reading, 135, 169
Nuances and cycle of remedy, 39
Nudity at home, yet shy and proper in company, 160
Numbness, 27, 31
Nurse, inability to, due to ulcerated throat, 150
Nurturance, 30, 33
*Nux vomica*, 151-152

Obedience, after remedy, 87
Obedience, see also Disobedience
Object of fear vs. effect of fear, 43, 55
Objects destroyed, 113
Objects, shiny, fear of, in meningitis, 171
Oblivious to pain, 137
Obnoxious behavior, 29, 154
Observing joy of violence, 85
Obsession over women's breasts, 160
Obsession with sexual matters, 160
Obsessive behavior, 46, 51, 78, 109, 112
Obstinacy, 12, 73, 79, 98, 109
Obviousness to presence, 108
Occiput, as locus of headache, 136
Occult preoccupations, 66
Ocean, fear of, 65, 148
Off balance of vital force, 6

Offense imagined, 77
Old brain, hypothalamus and limbic system, 34-35
Older children, and advice on night terrors, 125
Opisthotonic posture in sleep, 132
Opisthotonos, 138, 162, 168
*Opium*, 16
Oppositional behavior, 83
Optometry, Behavioral, 140
Orange juice, craves, 156
Oranges, craves, 156
*Organon*, by Samuel Hahnemann, 181-186
*Organon*, aphorism 153 discussed, 4
*Origanum*, 94
Orphan, created by war of contradictions, 114
Otitis media and autism, 112
Otitis media, serous, 145
Outside, fear of, 66
Overcontrol, 108, 158
Overcontrol by child and night terrors, 125
Overcontrol by child see also Guarding, Vigilance, and Hypervigilance, 125
Overheating and seizures, 167
Overreaction segment of *Stramonium* and fevers, 164
Overreaction to violence, 74
Overreaction, violent, 11, 27
Oversensitive to pain, 137
Overshooting and overcorrection of vital force, 8, 27
Overshooting, desire to close off, 31
Overstimulation limited by confined spaces, 63
Overwhelmed feeling, 47, 79, 101

Pain as if being tortured, 177
Pain of headache drives child mad, 136
Pain, better touch, 13
Pain, fear of, 112
Pain, surrender to, 61
Painlessness of normally painful symptoms, 31, 137, 176
Pajama changing in night terrors with urination, 129
Palliation of talking and psychotherapy, 54
Pampered, feeling of being, 58
Panic in night terror, 123
Panic, 43, 49, 60, 67, 76, 98

Panthers, fear of, 59
Paradoxical nature of fears, 56
Paralyzed by fear, 45, 54
Paralyzed from fear of water in eyes, 64
Paralyzed psychically, 106
Parent as monster, 122
Parent may die, fear that, 66
Parent refuses to talk to child, 177
Parent returning to work, abandonment and ear infections, 145
Parent/child link, establishing in night terrors, 129
Parent/child relationship shaken by bedtime war, 118
Parental changes as child improves, 101
Parental response to night terrors, 124-126
Parents aggravate night terrors inadvertently, 124
Parents different from him, causes fear, two year old, 176
Parents or others not recognized, 32, 76
Parents, sleeping with child, 58
Passageway between conscious and unconscious opened by naming triggers of night terrors, Step 4, 126
Passions and logic, 19
Passions unleashed, 34
Passions, remedies ruled by, 20
Pasta, craves, 21
Pathological states, intensity of, 16
Pathology level, 27
Pathology of *Stramonium* compared with nosodes and polychrests, 38
Patient history, birth trauma and eye problems, 140
Pattern of shock, injury and abandonment, 177
Pattern of symptoms, 28
Pattern of night terrors, things to break it, 120
Patterns and behavior with both sleep and waking state, 121
Patterns, 9, 13
Peculiar symptoms, 39
Peers consider her weird, 135
Penis held, in Tourette's syndrome, 170
Penis, 160
Penis, holding incessantly, 149
Penis, holding, when frightened, 170
People as animals or other beings or things, 32

People, adverse to, 172
People, fear of, 48, 53, 59
Perceptions altered, 113
Perfectionism, 95, 113
Perpetual fear, 44
Perseverative behavior, 78, 93, 98, 108-111, 110, 112, see also Ritual and unrelenting behavior
Personality change in encephalitis, 172
Personality changes after head injuries, 135, 136
Perspiration, especially head and upper torso in sleep, 132
Perspiration, profuse, 29
Perspiration, scalp, 21
Perspiration, scanty, except during sleep, 164
Pertussis vaccine, see DPT
Pertussis, 150, 151
Peter Rabbit, 68, 81
Petite mal, 167
Phase four, 17, 21, 22
Phase four, two categories of, 20
Phase one, 19, 21-23, 35
Phase three, 17, 19-22
Phase two, 19, 21, 22, 35
Phases, *Stramonium's* place in, 34-35
Phimosis, 160
*Phosphorus*, 16, 151-152
Photophobia in fevers, 163
Photophobia, 60, 141
Physical abuse, 61
Physical developmental delays, 109
Physical generals, 23
Physical symptoms of *Stramonium* not well known, 38
Physical symptoms, general, 174-177
Picked on, fear of being, 43
Picky eater, 156
Picture as ghost, 122
*Pierre*, by Herman Melville, 117
Pies, 12
Pigmentation, loss of, compensating for inner darkness, 165
Pinned down in bed, delusion of, in fever, 164
Pins, fear of, xi
Plants amputates, 83
Plastic, smelling of, 111
*Platina*, 16, 81
Play, aversion to, 166

Play, difficulties with, 71, 72, 78
Playful aspect of stare, 139
Playground, behavior, 62
Plethoric appearance, 148
Pneumonia and loss of language skills, 97
Pneumonia, 152-153
Pneumonia, dry nose, initial heat phase, 146
Poetry, violent, 103
Polarity of aggression and inwardness, 43
Polarity of life and death, see Life and death
Policeman types, 80-81
Polychrest and miasms bridged, 14
Polychrests and *Hyoscyamus*, 20
Polychrests, 18, 19, 20, 37, 38
Polychrests, not fitting today's cases, xiii
Population of children vs. individual child, 17
Possessed, as if, 84, 100, 139
Post traumatic stress disorder, 101
Post-adrenal depression, 31
Potential disease, 17
Potter, Beatrix, 81
Pounding head in headache, 136
Power pack, blinding spray, 54
Powerless feeling of parent watching night terror, 124, 127
Precision, strived for, 112
Predatory sexuality, 162
Predicting symptoms, 12
Preemptive strike, 45
Pregnancy and baby after cured lymphoma, xi
Pregnancy predisposes child to *Stramonium*, 173
Pregnancy with fright predisposes child to *Stramonium* state, 174
Pregnancy, 69
Pregnancy, fright during, 65, 107
Pregnancy, frights during, causes *Stramonium* state in child, 173-174
Pregnancy, unwanted, 60
Pregnancy, vomiting in, 70
Premenstrual symptoms, 161
Presentiment of death, 33, 67
Pressing fingers into head in headaches, 136
Preventive care, homeopathically, 27
Prisoner, tortured in jail, as if, from pain, 144
Professional homeopaths and asthma, 155
Promiscuity, 162

Pronouncing letters difficult, as L, M, and W.
Protection, need of, 28, 30, 52
Protection, lack of, 177
Protective mechanism, 84
Proud, happy child in toilet training after remedy, 158
Proust, Marcel, 115
Proving of violent and darker aspects, 39
*Psorinum*, 16
Psyche, 99
Psyche, divided, 44, see also Consciousness/unconsciousness
Psychiatric medications, intense use of, 37
Psychic space intruded into by water, 64
Psychically protecting self, 106
Psychotherapy, 54
Public educational television, 52
Puckering, 82
Pulls hair, 172
*Pulsatilla*, xi, 16, 17, 142, 149
Punching in night terror, 123
Punching, 73, 79, 83, 102
Punishing behavior by child, 80
Punishment as non-issue, 49
Punishment, 120
Punishment for night terrors increases night terrors, 121
Punishment, no fear of, 84
Pupils, dilate, 84, 139
Puppet shows, 52
Purposeful restlessness, 91
Purposelessness, 91
Pus in eyes, 142
Push-pull existence, 95
Push-pull scenario, nightly, 117
Pushing, 47, 83
Pyelonephritis and pregnant mother, 173

Questioning children lovingly in night terrors, 128
Questions ignored, appears not to hear, 81, 97, 145
Quiet, 100
Quiet, during fever, 52

Rage, 45, 73, 74, 76, 79, 84, 89, 102, 139
Rage, expressed in sexuality due to past abuse, 162
Rain, enjoyed or may aggravate, 175

Rambunctious, 52
Random discharge of energy, 75
Rare and peculiar symptoms, 13
Rash, skin, 164
Rashes, lower abdomen and groin area, 165
Rationale behind violence, 45, 80
Rats, 53
Ravaged by monsters, dreams of, 161
Reactive, xi
Reactivity, 77-80, 92
Read, desire to, 87
Read, inability to, 96
Reading horror novels, 135
Reading, same book every night, 118
Reality and dreams confused, 120
Reality confused, 27, 31, 76
Realm of death vs. life realm, 32
Reason, gift of, 34
Reasoning, defined, 19
Reclusive premenstrually, 161
Rectum, 158-159
Red eyes, 142
Red face with fever and earache, 143
Regression since surgery, 96
Regression to baby state, 153
Regression, 74
Relentlessness, 94
Relation of symptoms, 13-14
REM sleep, 120
Remedies, effect of, in autism, 105, 114
Remedy groups, differentiating, 16
Remedy layers, 19
Remedy, effect of, 67, 86-88
Remedy, effect of, on impetigo and emotional concomitants, 166
Remedy, not given in favor of nourishment and not interfering with healing process, 155
Remedy, wrong, prescribed, 88
Remorse magnified by sleep, 115
Renal failure and pregnant mother, 173
Repatterning of visual skills, 140
Repercussions of actions understood, 86
Repercussions vs. immediate survival, 48
Repertory, ear infections and *Stramonium*, 142-143
Repetitive actions, 93
Repression of abuse addressed by remedy, 161-162

Reprimands and stammering, 146
Respiratory infection in dentition, 146
Respiratory tract infections and fevers, 163
Respiratory tract infections, importance of, in bodies' health, 154
Restful sleep after remedy in night terror, 131
Restlessness and hyperactivity, 89
Restlessness with violence and acting out, 84
Restlessness in autism, 112
Restlessness, 81, 82, 89, 90, 175
Restlessness, constant state of, 90
Restraint, causing violence, 75
Retching in the morning, 156
Retreat into inner world, 61-62, 113
Retreat, desire to, 30
Retreating to fetal position, 61
*Rhus toxicodendron* and *Lycopodium* compared in arthritis, 23
Ribs feel bruised, 152
Right eye staring, left eye involuntarily closed, 141
Right lower side and left upper side, rashes, 164
Right sided symptoms of lower body, 175
Rigid actions, 118
Rigidity and water, 63, 64
Rigidity in seizures, 168
Rigidity of will, 93
Rigidity when held, 90
Rigidity with fright, 56
Rigidity, 48, 65
Ripping through barrier of consciousness/ unconsciousness, 34, 43
Rips own clothes, 86
Ritual abuse, 145
Ritualism as self-abusive behavior, 106
Ritual broken, 78
Ritualistic behavior from reaction to hives, 165
Ritualistic and unrelenting behavior, 45, 46, 93, 105, 106, 108-111, 110, 118, 156
Ritualistic behavior, reasoning behind, 109
Ritualistic behavior, two sides of, 109
Rocking convulsively, 169
Rocking, 48, 81, 82, 94, 108
Rolling head side to side, arms flailing without control, 169
Rolling on ground in headache, 136
Rolling, 76
Roseola, 52

Rothenberg, Amy, 37
Rubbed, desire to be, 12
Rubric, 62, 79
Rubrics and segment, 11
Rudeness as control mechanism, 72
Rules, 51
Running, 54
Rushing behavior, 90

Sadistic look, 172
Sadness, 72, 101
Safe environment and arresting of autism, 107
Safety, feeling of, after remedy in night terror, 130
Sailor thrown by cruel wave on shores of light, as if, 174
Salami, craves, 156
Salem, Massachusetts, witch trial museum, 51
Salt, craved, 156
Sandy sensation in eyes, 142
Scared, 153
Schizophrenic break, 60
School scene and restlessness, 90
School work, loses, 94
Science fiction, 38
Scratched face, appears like wild animal, 165
Scratches parents in night terror, 123
Scratching and severe infections, 165
Scratching face during nightmare, 166
Scratching in seizure, 76, 168
Scratching, 74, 75, 78, 79, 92
Screaming and vaccinations, 176
Screaming in meningitis, 171
Screaming in night terror, 123, 124
Screaming, 45, 48, 54, 58, 70, 72, 76, 77, 78, 79, 80, 81, 112, 117, 144
Secluded, 100
Seesaw war of life/death, conscious/unconsciousness, 34
Segments, fundamental, in cycle, 9-13
Segments of *Stramonium* cycle, 28-32
Segments, 10, 11
Seizure and wrinkled forehead, 148
Seizure in ear inflammation, 144
Seizure while showering, 172
Seizure, as if in, when stammering, 146
Seizures and back problems, 162
Seizures and DPT vaccine, 176
Seizures and eye rolling, 140

Seizures and vaccines, 176
Seizures in infections, 149
Seizures in sleep, 132
Seizures, 29, 30, 63, 66, 76, 89, 113, 135, 138, 140, 166-169, 174, 175
Seizures and red face, 147
Seizures, febrile, 163
Seizures following antipathic treatment of eczema, 164
Seizures in dentition, 146
Seizures, many daily, since encephalitis, 172
Seizures, mild, resembling shivering and teeth chattering, 167
Seizures, triggered by terror, 50
Seizures, weakness following, 31
Self absorbed, so injury not felt, 137
Self and reality confused, 76
Self blame, 55, 102
Self concept, poor, 99
Self directed violence, 85-86
Self esteem, 100
Self hatred, 102, 103
Self importance, lack of, in suicidal attitude, 103
Self preservation instinct, lack of, 67
Self-abusive behavior, 106
Sensitive, xi, 72
Senses acute, 55
Sensory input overload, 77
Sensory integration 77-79
Sensory integration difficulties, 98
Sensory/motor development delayed, 112
Sentence formation after taking remedy, 114
Sentences, lovingly and calmly spoken in night terrors calm child, 128
Sentences, stuck in the middle of, 146
Sentimental, xi
Separation from parents, feared, 102
Separation of parents, 108
Separation, fear of, 116
Sequalae of ear infections, 142
Sequence in an illness: horrors, infolded personality, aggression, infection, fear of pain, overreaction, closing off, 112
Sequence in introversion: impulsiveness, guilt over impulsiveness, control of impulses, hyper vigilance, shutting down, 117
Sequence of sleep pathology: wakes confused, fears develop, moves to escape fear, overreacts in violence, closes off, shuts down, 131

Sequential progression to terror from inability to speak, 113
Severe nausea and vomiting and *Stramonium* state, 174
Sex drive high, 162
Sexual abuse, 61, 161
Sexual acting out, 94
Sexual behavior premenstrually, 161
Sexual joking, 96
Sexual language, 160
Shadows, 50, 67
Shaking of child in night terror aggravates, 124
Shame over actions, 101
Sharks in dreams, 121
Shaving cream, playing with , 112
Shell, coming out of, 79
Shell-shocked, 99
Shipping cartons, fear of, 62
Shock from injury as etiology, 177
Shoelaces, tying, 78
Shoes as play lethal weapon, 85
Shower, hot, and seizures, 167
Showers, fear of, 63, 119
Shrieking in headache, 136
Shrieking of child in night terrors, 124
Shrieking, 49, 58, 59, 74, 80, 90
Shutting down, 25, 31, 75, 102, 103, 105, 108, see also Death and deadness
Shyness, xi, 43
Siblings, hurt, as reaction to parents anger with them, 80
Side, buried alive, delusion of, 62
Sidedness of rashes, 164
Sidedness of *Stramonium* in earache and fever, 143-145
Sidedness of symptoms, 175
Sidedness, left or right handed, developmentally delayed, 163
Sign language, 113
Sign of parental contact established in night terrors is deep breathing, 128
Silly behavior and vertigo, 138
Silly behavior, 93
Similar states and remedy selection, 15
Similarities vs. differences, 12
Simultaneous sleep and waking state, 121
Sister eaten by a big dog in night terror, 122
Sits still, cannot, 158

Sitting close to child in night terrors, 125
Skin eruptions suppressed as etiology in nervous system disturbances, 171
Skin eruptions, suppression of, as etiology, 177
Skin pigment, loss of, 165
Skin, 164-166
Skin, gouging own, 85
Skin, red, chafing, 148
Slaps do not waken from night terror, 123
Sleep aggravation times, midnight and 2 a.m., 132
Sleep difficulties, 90
Sleep position, 7, 132
Sleep stage, stuck in, 114
Sleep symptoms, general, 116, 132-133
Sleep with light on, 51
Sleep, 57, 154
Sleep, aggravations in, 175
Sleep, as if warded off, in meningitis, 172
Sleep, drifting off, 115
Sleep, fear of, 120
Sleep, fears before, 116-119
Sleep, intrusion on, 73
Sleep, missing, aggravates, 176
Sleep, non-REM, 121
Sleep, poor in heat, 175
Sleep, REM, 120
Sleep, restless, 132
Sleep, screaming in, 70
Sleep, symptoms, general 132
Sleep, transition from REM to non-REM and night terrors, 121
Sleeping alone, fear of, 119
Sleeping by self after remedy in night terror, 130
Sleeping in and going to bed late, after head injury, 135
Sleeping with parents, 58, 79, 118, 119
Sleepwalking, 132
Slides, fear of, 62
Sliding out of chair in encephalitis, 172
Smacking herself, 86
Smacking, 66
Smell, loss of, 31
Smells, finicky about, 111
Smiling in seizure, 168
Smoke aggravates asthma, 176
Smoking *Stramonium*, 39
Snakes, fear of, 51, 53

Social skills, missing, 99
Socializing, 51
*Sodomme et Gomorrhe*, by Marcel Proust, 115
Soldier, like a lone, retreating, 100
*Solve Your Child's Sleep Problems*,
   by Richard Ferber
Somatized fear and abdominal
   complaints, 158
Sorrow magnified by sleep, 115
Soul ripped from body, as if, 123, 139
Soul, beyond conscious ego, 120
Soul, fear, loss of, 51
Soul, mystery of, 117
Sound as relaxant, 58
Sounds as wild animals, 122
Sounds, weird, everywhere in dreams, 124
Spaces out, 97
Spasmodic cough in asthma, 153
Spasmodic cough, 150
Spasms of throat, 149
Spasms, 29, 30
Spasms, benign, infantile, 168
Speaking, seems to, in meningitis, 171
Speaks of killing self, 95
Spectator sport, view of life, 100
Specters, 50
Speech difficulty, compensated for by
   writing skills, 113
Speech improved after remedy, 67, 97
Speech, ability lost, 96, 113
Speech, baby talk, 96
Speech, developmentally delayed, 112
Speech, fast, 53, 61
Speech, gender mistakes in, 96
Speech, lost and regained, 114
Speech, loud, 94
Speech, rapid and sucking up air, 146, 170
Speech, staccato, 113
Speech, stammering, 146
Spider web of heightened neural activity, 79
Spider webs in dreams, 124
Spinal tap in meningitis aggravates
   *Stramonium* state, 144
Spinal tap, 70
Spiral downward in disease, 9
Spiral downward of pathology, 27
Spiritual enlightenment, 60
Spiritual support of life processes lacking, 34
Spits, 79, 172

Spitting words, 61
Spitting on parents, 84, 91
*Spongia tosta*, 151-152
Spots on skin, red and itchy, 165
Spring tightly compressed as *Stramonium*
   comparison, 73
Squinting, 141
Squirming, 91
Stages of illness in remedy picture, 7
Stages of pathology, 27
Stages of violence, 84
Stammering with jerking motions, 170
Stammering, 29, 33, 140, 146, 147
Strangers, 177
Staphylococcal infections, 165
*Staphysagria*, 55, 100, 101, 148
Stare, autistic, 139
Staring as if dead, 139
Staring in meningitis, 171
Staring in night terror, 127
Staring in seizures, 168
Staring, 71, 108, 148, 169
Startled to half wakefulness, 118
Starvation, in earlier life, and voracious
   appetite, 155
Statues, weird, in dreams, 124
Status epilepticus, 172
Step one to four in eliminating night
   terrors, 126-129
Sternocleidomastoid contracts causing
   neck pain, 163
Sternum, ribs feel as if separating from, 152
Steroids and development of
   neurodermatitis, 165
Stimuli as mirror of inner turmoil, 44
Stimuli of night terrors, exposure to
   diminished, (Step 3) 126
Stimuli overload, 93
Stomach aches, 157-158
Stomach, 155-157
Stomping, 79
Stool, scanty in fevers, 163
Stools loose from sweets, 156
Stools, involuntary, 159
Stools, loose, 142, 158-159
Stools, mucousy, xi
Stools, solid, after remedy, 158
Stories, good and evil, limiting, 68
Stories, scary, 119, 160

Strabismus, convergent, 140
Strabismus, surgery and meningitis, 171, 177
Strain to adjust stress, 6
Strains shown by vital force, 8, 11, 181-186
Straits of *Stramonium*, isthmus between conscious/unconsciousness, 34-35
*Stramonium*, *Hyoscyamus* compared by symptom intensity level, 17
*Stramonium*, differentiating, *Calcarea*, *Tuberculinum*, *Veratrum*, 20-21
*Stramonium* ameliorates Tourette's syndrome, 170
*Stramonium* and *Arnica montana* compared, 48
*Stramonium* and *Calcarea carbonica* compared in night terrors, 122
*Stramonium* and *Hyoscyamus* compared in attention difficulties, 92
*Stramonium* and *Hyoscyamus* compared, 50
*Stramonium* and *Lyssinum* compared in self violence, 85
*Stramonium* and *Medorrhinum* compared as layers, 87
*Stramonium* and *Natrum muriaticum* compared in suicidal thoughts, 103
*Stramonium* and *Sulphur*, example of suppression, 88
*Stramonium* as complementary with *Natrum muriaticum* and *Staphysagria*, 101
*Stramonium* as confused with nosodes and polychrests, 38
*Stramonium* as overprescribed and underprescribed, 38
*Stramonium* camouflaged as polychrest, nosode, or mania remedy, 37
*Stramonium* compared to *Belladonna* in headache, behavior and intensity, 137
*Stramonium* compared to *Medorrhinum* in problem of extremities, 163
*Stramonium* compared with *Medorrhinum* in bowel complaints, 158
*Stramonium* cycle exemplified in night terror, 131
*Stramonium* compared to *Hyoscyamus* in sexuality, 160, 162
*Stramonium* compared in headaches: *Chamomilla*, *Lachesis*, *Tarentula hispanica*, *Lycopodium*, 136
*Stramonium* compared to *Belladonna* in red facial coloring, 147-148

*Stramonium* compared to *Tuberculinum*, *Veratrum album*, *Tarantula hispanica*, *Lachesis*, in destructive behavior, 82
*Stramonium* compared with *Helleborus* and *Tuberculinum* in head rolling, hitting, 138
*Stramonium* compared with *Apis mellifica* in dehydrating fever, 159
*Stramonium* compared with *Arsenicum album*, *Belladonna* in earache and fever, 143
*Stramonium* compared with *Belladonna*, *Pulsatilla*, *Sulphur* in sore throats, 149
*Stramonium* compared with *Belladonna*, *Spongia tosta*, *Drosera*, *Nux vomica*, *Phosphorus* in respiratory symptoms, 151-152
*Stramonium* compared with *Bryonia alba* in pneumonia, 152-153
*Stramonium* compared with *Helleborus* and *Hyoscyamus* in meningitis, 172
*Stramonium* compared with *Hyoscyamus*, *Lachesis* in throat spasms and constrictions, 149
*Stramonium* compared with *Hyoscyamus* in hyperactivity, 84
*Stramonium* compared with *Hyoscyamus* in involuntary movement, 169
*Stramonium* compared with *Hyoscyamus* in involuntary stools, 159
*Stramonium* compared with *Hyoscyamus* in joking, 96
*Stramonium* compared with *Hyoscyamus* in Tourette's syndrome, 170
*Stramonium* compared with *Lachesis* and *Hyoscyamus* in loquacity, 96
*Stramonium* compared with *Lycopodium* and *Baryta carbonica* in undescended testicle, 160
*Stramonium* compared with *Lycopodium* in ritual manipulation, 109
*Stramonium* compared with *Lycopodium* in wrinkling of forehead, 148
*Stramonium* compared with *Medorrhinum*, *Euphrasia*, *Pulsatilla*, *Sulphur* in eye infections, 142.
*Stramonium* compared with *Natrum muriaticum* and *Staphysagria* in introversion, 100
*Stramonium* compared with *Natrum muriaticum* and *Staphysagria*, 55
*Stramonium* compared with *Sulphur* and *Tuberculinum* in loose stools, 158
*Stramonium* compared with *Sulphur* in eczema, 164-165

*Stramonium* compared with *Sulphur*, *Medorrhinum* and *Veratrum album* in food cravings and aversions, 157
*Stramonium* compared with *Tarantula hispanica* and *Hyoscyamus* in arrogance, 84
*Stramonium* compared with *Tarantula hispanica* in rocking, 169
*Stramonium* compared with *Tuberculinum, Cina, Chamomilla, Sulphur* in dentition, 146-147
*Stramonium* compared with *Tuberculinum* in teeth grinding, 132
*Stramonium* compared with *Veratrum album* and *Tarantula hispanica* in touching everything, 90
*Stramonium* compared with *Medorrhinum* in sleep positions, 132
*Stramonium* compared with *Staphysagria* in facial tics, 148
*Stramonium* cycle, 27-36, 122
*Stramonium* essence sentence, 8
*Stramonium* layer and sexual abuse,161
*Stramonium* needed by mother, 173
*Stramonium* pathology preceding onset of Tourette's, 170
*Stramonium* similar to *Lycopodium* in torticollis, 163
*Stramonium* similar to *Natrum muriaticum, Calcarea carbonica, Tuberculinum* in food cravings, 156
*Stramonium* compared with *Hyoscyamus*, and *Medorrhinum*, and symptom intensities, 18
*Stramonium*, hallucinogenic effects of, 39
*Stramonium*, shared symptoms with *Tuberculinum* and *Lycopodium*, 21
*Stramonium, Tuberculinum, Hyoscyamus* compared, 80
*Stramonium, Veratrum album, Tarantula hispanica, Hyoscyamus, Platina*, as haughty remedies, 81
*Stramonium, Veratrum album, Tarantula hispanica* and *Lachesis* as whirlwind of energy remedies, 113
Strangers, fear of, 47, 49, 50
Streptococcal infection and encephalitis, 172
Streptococcal infection, 52, 54, 152, 165
Streptococcal infection, headache and temporary blindness, 141
Stress of day, surfacing at night, 116
Stress trigger of night terror recognized, 127
Stress, 98, 126

Stress, emotional, during day, expressed as fears of bedtime, 120
Stress, slight, causes overload, 78
Stresses and triggers of night terrors identified (step 1), 126
Stresses, internal in origin, 117
Striking, 30, 72, 76, 84, 94
Strings, holding him down, 164
Stroke pain similar to headache, 136
Stroke symptoms in organic brain disease, 135
Stubborn, 66
Stuck between sleep and waking, 122
Stuck thought acted out, 78
Study, inability to, 97
Stuffed nose, obstructing breathing, 146
Stuttering, 97
Subarachnoid hemorrhages, 174
Subdued state, 101
Suffocating, as if, 62, 154
Suicidal tendency, 55
Suicide, 102, 103
Sullen, 100
*Sulphur*, 16, 88, 142, 146-147, 149, 156-157, 158
Sun, aspects of, aversion to, 175
Sunlight reflected and violence or panic, 60
Sunlight reflected on glass, 141
Sunstrokes, 175
Superhero, dressing as, 160
Supernatural forces, 50
Supportive, loving adults, 61
Suppressed violence and teen years, 86
Suppression, 88
Suppression, classic definition of, 23
Surgery as etiology of meningitis, 171
Surgery as etiology, 177
Surgery, 96
Surroundings, unaware of, 94
Survival, 64
Susceptibility to diseases from sexual abuse, 162
Susceptibility, 39
Suspiciousness, 14
Suturing of consciousness and unconsciousness by remedy in night terrors, 130
Swaddled excessively, 56
Swaddling, fear of, 62
Swaggering and vertigo, 138
Swallowing, painful, 149

Swamps in dreams, 124
Sweet with cats, mean with kids, 86
Sweet during fever, 52
Sweet disposition after remedy, 87
Sweets and ear infections, 145
Sweets and hyper behavior, 176
Sweets and recurring coughs, 151
Sweets, 12
Sweets, craves, xi, 10, 13, 142, 156
Swelling of penis, 160
Swim, learning to, 63, 65
Swimming pool chills and *Stramonium* coughs, 151
Swimming, 126
Swimming, learning how and seizures, 171
Swinging, 82
Swords, obsession with, 78, 110
Symbols of death, 31
Symptom intensity, 38
Symptomology shared by *Stramonium* in map of hierarchy, 37
Symptoms and segments, 11-13
Symptoms in brain disease, 135
Symptoms, 3
Symptoms, divergent, coexisting, 67
Symptoms, most limiting, 24
Symptoms, most striking, 4
Symptoms, new, produced by remedy, 59
Symptoms, overfocusing on, as opposed to those representing the individual, 170
Symptoms, severe, as priority, 87
Symptoms, sleep, necessary for confirming remedy, 115
Symptoms, to discover reason behind, 98
Systems dynamics of addiction loop, 29, 65

Tachypnea, 174
Tactile defensiveness, 112
Talking in seizure, 168
Talking in sleep, 132
Talking with child about trigger fears of night terrors before bed, 127
Tantrums as method of dealing with the unexpected, 80
*Tarentula hispanica*, 16, 81, 82, 84, 90, 113, 136, 169
*Tarentulas*, 53
Tattoos on arms, 169
Taunted, 43

Tearing at people in seizures, 168
Tearing of consciousness/unconsciousness barrier, 34
Tearing, 30, 79, 91
Tears in infections, 142
Teasing cough, 150
Teasing, 160
Teenagers and controlled violence, 86
Teenagers, 57, 100
Teeth grinding cured in night terror, 131
Teeth grinding in meningitis, 172
Teeth grinding in seizures, 168
Teeth grinding, 90, 102, 132, 146, 152
Teeth, 146-147
Television violence, 84, 119
Television, 38
Television, limiting, 68
Television, too real, 51
Temper tantrum, 51, 71, 72, 78, 79, 80, 82, 85, 86, 95, 110, 113, 137, 153
Temper tantrums and headaches, 136
Temples, as locus of headache, 136
Temporal lobe epilepsy, 106, 168
Temporal lobe, EEG changes, 113
Tense and taught in fevers, 164
Tension in sleep, 125
Terrified of death, 28
Terror magnified by sleep, 115
Terror of repeating dreams, 116
Terror, 29, 49, 54, 61, 65, 70, 100, 106, 113, 116, 122, 139
Terror erupting out of chronic fear, 45
Terror, programming scenario to affect, 106
Testicles, undescended, 160
*The Meaning of Psychology for Modern Man*, by Carl Jung, 120
*The Prince*, by Niccolo Machiavelli, 109
Thirsty and thirstless, 156
Thirsty, cold drinks, 142
Thomas, Dylan, 69
Thoracic pain, 13
Thoughts, automatically voiced in Tourette's syndrome, 170
Thoughts, morbid, 103
Thrashing head on pillow, 76
Thrashing in night terror, 122, 123, 124
Thrashing, 59
Threatened miscarriage in first trimester and *Stramonium* state, 174

Threatening attitude construed by child, 107
Threatening, 71, 73
Threats and violent rituals to control others, 109
Threats in dreams, 121
Threshold of fear, 54
Thrill of violence, mimicked, to vent fears, 81
Throat infection, 54
Throat ulcers, 150
Throat, 149-150
Throat, paralysis of, 149
Throat, rough and dry, feels, 149
Throbbing in ears, 143
Throwing self on ground, 102
Throwing things, 47, 74, 49, 83
Thrown into water, learning to swim, and seizures, 171
*Thuja*, 16
Thunder and lightning enjoyed, 175
Thunderstorms, fear of, 51, 54, 65, 66
Tics in Tourette's syndrome, 170
Tics, 89, 148
Tics following antipathic treatment of eczema, 164
Tigers, 53, 66
Time aggravation, 2 a.m., 144
Time aggravations, midnight and 2 a.m., 175
Time-bomb of bedtime, 118
Timid normally yet violent in seizures, 168
Timid, xi
*To the Arms of the Sea*, by Jeenet Lawson, 99
Toddlers, masturbation in, 94
Toilet bowl monster, 53
Toilet training, 66, 112, 158
Tolerance, lack of, 78
Tomatoes and canker sores, 147
Tomatoes and tomato sauce, aversion to, 156
Tongue, 146
Tonic clonic seizure, 168
Tonsillitis accompanied by fever and sharp pain, 149
Torn to pieces, fear of being, 53
Torticollis, 163
Torture, 44, 45, 48, 50, 68, 82, 84, 116, 143, 145
Tossing in sleep, 90, 132
Total pattern of a disease, 8
Totality of remedy and person, 4, 7
Totality of symptoms and unit of disease, 6

Totality of symptoms, 8
Touch aggravates, 78
Touch as intrusion, 73
Touch triggering night terrors, 121
Touch, as pain, 48
Touch, aversion, to, 74
Touch, sensitivity to, 12
Touches everything, 83, 90
Touching head before seizures, 138
Touching objects, 112
Tough kids, 63
Tourette's syndrome, 76
Toy rituals, 109
Toying with innocent people, 139
Toys, 92
Toys, destroys, 82, 83
Train travel as similar to disease cycles, 9
Trance-like state, 97, 109
Transition, critical, to common world, 102
Transitional remedies, 14, 19
Trapped, fear of being, 62, 63
Trauma and attention difficulties, 96
Trauma to brain as etiology in autism, 108
Trauma to brain and seizures, 138
Tree with spider webs in dreams, 124
Trees, fright in, 56
Trigger stimuli of night terrors named, 126
Trigger, stimuli, 33, 43
Trip, reaction to, 90-91
Truth, realizing an alarming, 106
Tube in playground, 62
Tubercular side of *Stramonium*, 159
*Tuberculinum*, 16, 20, 40, 82, 117, 132, 138, 146-147, 154, 156, 158
*Tuberculinum*, shared symptoms with *Stramonium* and *Baryta carbonica*, 20
*Tuberculinum*, going to *Stramonium* after fright, 22
Tug of war, 33, 44, 122
Tug of war of desires, 30
Tunnels, fear of, 62
Turning in sleep, 132
Turning point in homeopathy, 14
Twin, fraternal, 124
Twitches, facial or extremities in fever, 163
Twitching around eyelids, 139
Twitching in sleep, 132
Twitching, 12, 63, 76, 91, 170

Two minds, as if, 32
Two years of age, symptoms begin to be exhibited, 176
Tympanic membrane, red, 143

Ulceration of throat, 150
Umbilical cord around neck as etiology, 107
Umbilical cord wrapped around neck, 174
Unconscious seems possessed, 168
Unconscious violence, 77
Unconscious world, 75
Unconscious, 57
Unconsciousness erupting into consciousness, 130
Unconsciousness, supreme reign of, 35
Unconsciousness, containment breached by sleep, 118
Uncovers body in sleep, 132
Unfolding pattern of disease, 8
Uniqueness of remedy, 11
Unitary aspect of disease, 6,7
Universal language of study and practice, 7
Universality of understanding, 28
Universe of good, 40
Unpredictability in other kids, 77
Unrelenting behavior, 93-94, 154
Unsteady gait, 170
Untuned vital force, 6
Upper respiratory infections and fear, 52
Upper respiratory tract infection and pale face, 147
Upper respiratory tract infection and teeth grinding in sleep, 132
Upper respiratory tract infections, 66, 76, 147, 152
Upper respiratory tract infections, acute, and back problems, 162
Urinary system, 159
Urinate, inability to, 31
Urinating in sleep, triggering nightmares, 129
Urinating on floor in sleep,123, 132
Urination in sleep causing night terrors, 126-127
Urination profuse in toddlers at night, 159
Urination, 53
Urination, excessive, 29
Urination, scanty in fevers, 163
Urine flow increased or decreased, 159
Urine odorless and light color, 159
Urine, night, differentiation with other remedies, 159

Vaccination and autism, 108
Vaccination and meningitis symptoms, 70
Vaccination and strabismus, 140
Vaccination as etiology, 176
Vaccinations as etiology in nervous system disorders, 171
Vaccinations, 49, 140, 149, 150, 152
Vacuum extraction birth and *Stramonium* state, 174
Vacillation, 95
Vacuum cleaner, 49
Vaginal bleeding, 11
Validating daytime experiences before bedtime, 127
Vampire teenager, (parental description), 135
Vampires, 50
Vegetables, raw, craved, 156
Vegetables, craves, xi
Venturesome, 67
*Veratrum album*, 15, 16, 20, 81, 82, 90, 113, 156-157
Verbal ability, lack of, 113
Verbalize, inability to, 47
Verbalizing as door opener in night terrors, 130
Vertigo from high places, xi
Vertigo, 138-139
Video games discouraged to eliminate night terrors, 127
Video games, 38
Video's, 54
Videos, limiting, 68
Vigilance, tense, at night, 120
Vindictiveness, 81
Violated, fear of being, 116
Violence after head injuries, 135
Violence and desire for darkness, 60
Violence as reaction to intrusion on private world, 172-174
Violence as reaction to being offended, 172
Violence as reaction to fear, 74
Violence as unconscious reaction, 75-76
Violence at eighteen months, 174
Violence for the sake of violence, 30
Violence in fever delirium, 163
Violence mirrored in parents watching night terror, 125

Violence, stages and end results, 84
Violence with fear, 43
Violence without meanness, 75
Violence, progressive stages of, 84
Violence, xi, 15, 20, 23, 35, 37, 39, 45, 69-88, 89, 91, 94, 96, 98, 99, 100, 102, 103, 107, 109, 113, 119, 150, 153, 156, 157, 177
Violence, changed by repatterning visual skills, 140
Violence, conscious/unconscious and state between, 75
Violence, diminishes, 86
Violence, may be lacking in *Stramonium* picture, 112
Violence, pleasure in, see Joy of violence,
Violence, self inflicted, 102
Violent behavior and hives, 165
Violent behavior and sweets, 176
Violent behavior premenstrually, 161
Violent father's alcoholism of several generations, 174
Violent in seizures, 168
Violent overreaction segment, 25
Violent overreaction, 10, 11, 29-30, 54, 69, 76, 89, 91, 96
Violent rituals and control of others, 109
Viral infection, 151
Viral meningitis, 76
Virus, 3
Vision loss, 31
Visions, 106, 116
Visions, disturbing, 101
Visions, hideous, 118
Visualizing fears as real, 52
Vital force and overreaction, 29
Vital force, 6, 8, 11, 181-186
Vitalism, 67
Vitalistic philosophy vs. mechanical application, 7-9
Vithoulkas Expert System, xi
Vithoulkas, George, xi, 37, 119
Vitiligo, 165
Voice, hoarseness all winter, 150
Voices weird in dreams, 124
Vomit in sleep, 66
Vomiting and DPT vaccine, 176
Vomiting from cough, 144
Vomiting in pregnancy, 70
Vomiting, projectile, 156

Vulnerability kicks dormant fears into gear, 49
Vulnerability, 25, 27, 28, 32, 46, 47, 48

Waking and sleeping state, split between, 32
Waking from deep sleep and night terrors, 121
Waking from sleep in temporary blindness, 141
Waking in night cured, 131
Waking up in sleep, 132
Waking screaming with earache, 143
Walking in dark, vertigo from dark, 138
Walking in sleep, 132
Walking on balls of feet, 170
Wallpaper attacking him in fever, 164
War veteran, closed off, resembling, 101
Warm blooded child, 158
Warm or hot in sleep, 132
Warmth aggravates eye infections 142
Warmth aggravates headache, 137
Water and light, 141-142
Water element in dreams, 124
Water, 65, 67, 148
Water, cold on child in night terror, aggravates, 125
Water, cold, desires to be in, 175
Water, fear of, 63, 127, 141
Water, fear of, and bed wetting, 132
Water, fear of, in meningitis, 172
Water, forced to go into and seizures, 171
Water, cold, craves, 149, 156
Waves, fear of, 65
Wax museum, fear in, 51
Way of being sick, 7
Weak spot of individual, 6
Weakness as segment, 11
Weakness following seizures, 31
Weapons, obsession with, 78, 85
Weeps when admonished, 85
Weight loss, 152
Werewolves, 87
Wheat aggravates, red skin, 148
Wheezing and asthma, 153
Whimpers, 71
Whining in sleep, 132
Whining, 149
Whirlwind of energy felt in child's presence, 113
Whites of eyes glisten, 139
Whooping cough and pale face, 147

Whooping cough, 150
Why, of illness, 3
Why, the question of, 14
Wildness in meningitis, 138
Wildness, xi, 101, 108
Will power and battle of wills, 92
Wind, enjoyed, 175
Wind, howling, 50
Wind, may aggravate, 175
Winter months, of darkness, and fear, 58
Witch hunts, 51
Witch stories, 50
Witches, 52, 65, 109, 146, 168
Withdrawal from other children, 66
Withdrawal, 74, 100
Witnessing violence, 39
Wolf chewing heart in night terror, 122
Wolves in dreams, 121 149
Wolves, fear of, 53
Womb, darkness of, 56
Wool allergy and eczema, 165
Word and speech understood in sleep, 130
Words garbled, 61
Words heard, involuntary repetition of, 170
Words, making up, 95
Words, over reliance on, 35
Workaholic father, 174
Workaholic, 69
World view and fever, 52
World view and problem solving, 5
World view, unconscious filter, 44
World view, 19, 57
World view, internalized, 20
World, unaware of, in surrender to pain, 61
Wrinkled, forehead, 148
Wrists dangling limp, 83
Write, inability to, 98
Writes stories, bloody, creepy, and of defiling dead bodies, 135
Writing difficult, 72
Writing, transposing letters, 97

Yelling by parents in night terrors aggravates, 124
Yelling of parents as trigger for police behavior, 80
Yelling, 47, 59, 72
Yogurt, craves, 156
Younger than age, behavior seems, 95

Zest in case-taking, 5

# *About the Author*

Paul Herscu, N.D., a native of Rumania, is a graduate of the National College of Naturopathic Medicine, in Portland, Oregon. With his wife and partner Amy Rothenberg, N.D., and his children, Sophia, Misha, and Jonah, he resides in Amherst, Massachusetts, where he practices, teaches, and writes about homeopathy.

Dr. Herscu has taught widely throughout Europe and the United States. He is founder and director of the New England School of Homeopathy, and the editor of the pacesetting journal *The New England Journal of Homeopathy*. His first book, *The Homeopathic Treatment of Children: Pediatric Constitutional Types*, has been acclaimed as an exceptional description of eight well-known remedies as they relate specifically to children.